The Beautiful Old Tree

presents

CRVO Survivor

Healing Central Retinal Vein Occlusion

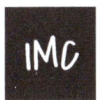

IMAGINE MEDIA CONCEPTS
FLORIDA

COPYRIGHT

CRVO Survivor:
Healing Central Retinal Vein Occlusion

Copyright © 2025 by The Beautiful Old Tree. All rights reserved. Published in the United States by Imagine Media Concepts.

Ebook ISBN: 979-8-9875354-8-6
Hardcover ISBN: 979-8-9923625-1-0
Paperback ISBN: 979-8-9923625-2-7
Audiobook ISBN: 979-8-9923625-0-3

Library of Congress Control Number: 2025900627

Imagine Media Concepts
Hollywood, FL 33020
www.imaginemediaconcepts.com

Cover Design by Imagine Media Concepts

LEGAL NOTICE:

Thank you for purchasing an authorized edition of this book and for complying with copyright laws by not reproducing or distributing this book without permission. Making or distributing electronic copies of this book constitutes copyright infringement and could subject the infringer to criminal and civil liability.

Licensed stock Images: Envato byrdyak, drazenphoto, and AdobeStock: 535480216, 965875373, 766632948, 535480216, 988419898. All other images, including patient images, are the property of Imagine Media Concepts and The Beautiful Old Tree.

DISCLAIMER NOTICE:

CRVO Survivor: Healing Central Retinal Vein Occlusion is brought to you by The Beautiful Old Tree, a website dedicated to collecting articles on health and well-being to promote happy and healthy aging.

www.thebeautifuloldtree.com

The author, who wishes to remain anonymous for personal reasons, is referred to as CRVO Survivor in the book. Any similarities to actual persons, living or deceased, are purely coincidental. The author and publisher disclaim any liability for any adverse effects resulting from the use of the information contained in this book.

From August 2024 to December 2024, Microsoft Copilot Pro was utilized throughout this book to provide research and reference material for the medical and technical information presented. Nearly all content includes links to the original medical websites from which the data was sourced. It has been an invaluable tool, helping to gather the necessary medical content, research, technical descriptions, and scientific data for this book.

Contents

INTRODUCTION

1. The Black Spot 1
2. My Story 5

CENTRAL RETINAL VEIN OCCLUSION

3. What is CRVO? 10
4. The Symptoms 22
5. What Causes it? 25
6. Known Treatments 30

PROFESSIONAL CARE

7. The Doctor's Visit 46
8. Injections 54
9. Laser Treatments 65
10. Vitrectomy Surgery 70

11. Complications. 74
12. After the Injection. 90
13. Follow-up Appointments 96

HEALING THE EYE

14. Is CRVO Curable?. 99
15. Exploring the Eye 103
16. John's Protocol 114

3 STEPS OF HEALING

17. The Game Plan 125
18. Step 1: Stop the Leak. 130
19. Step 2: Repair the Eye. 150
20. Step 3: Unblock the Blockage 184

FINAL THOUGHTS

21. Conclusion 214
22. Supplement Facts 227
23. Helpful Links. 234

CRVO Survivor

Healing Central Retinal Vein Occlusion

FOREWORD

This morning, I woke up to an email from a young man who had just been diagnosed with Central Retinal Vein Occlusion (CRVO). He was extremely frightened and didn't understand what was happening to him. His doctor, like mine, didn't offer many solutions. While searching the web for answers, he came across a post I had written years ago on a CRVO support group website about a protocol that helped me heal my eyesight. His email brought back the fear and helplessness I felt when I was first diagnosed with the disease.

For years, I've debated whether to write a book about my experience with CRVO because, after all, I am not a doctor, a medical professional, an ophthalmologist, or anyone of importance who has scientific knowledge on healing the eye. I am just a patient, a formally frightened patient at that, who, like millions of other

CRVO sufferers, has had to answer their own questions about Central Retinal Vein Occlusion and how to deal with the many problems and side effects that come along with the disease because either our doctors didn't know the answers to our questions or they didn't care enough to take the time to explain to us what was actually going on.

Because CRVO patients have few places to turn for answers, I've decided to share my story with the hope that it will help you in your healing process.

Best Wishes & Happy Healing
CRVO Survivor

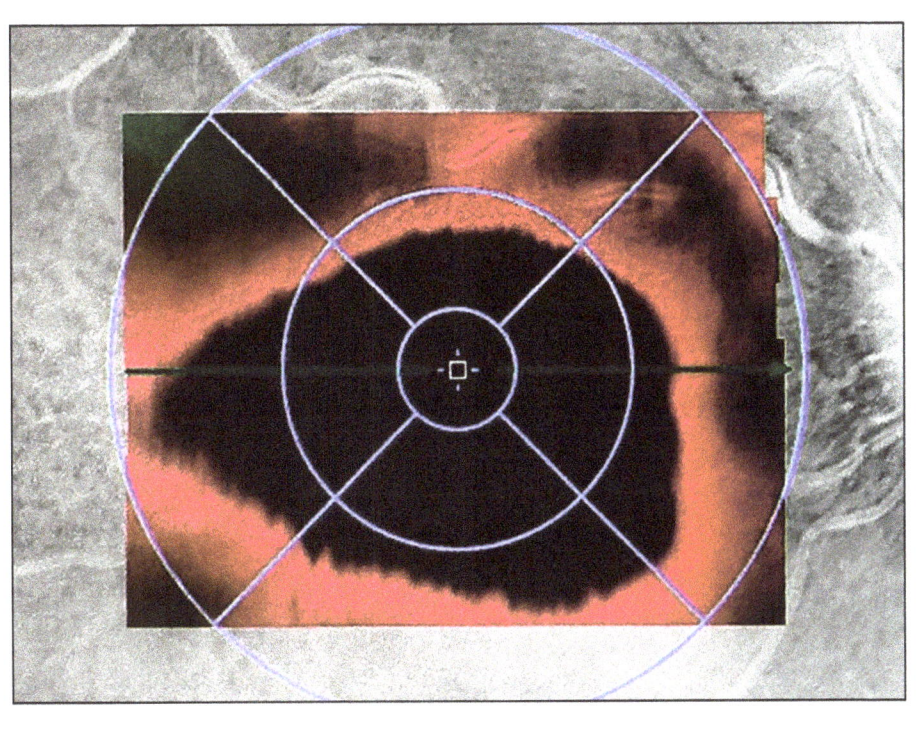

INTRODUCTION

1

The Black Spot

Have you ever wondered what life might have been like for Ludwig van Beethoven after he lost his hearing? It must have been terrifying. I can't imagine what he went through, knowing that music was the love of his life and that he wouldn't be able to hear it anymore.

For me, losing my vision would be similar to Beethoven's hearing loss. As a graphic designer and video editor, my world would stop if I lost my vision. The thought of losing my eyesight to Central Retinal Vein Occlusion was unacceptable to me. Despite the severity of my condition, I refused to believe that the body couldn't heal itself. From my first leakage until now, I have scrutinized every reaction to food, sleep, exercise, injections, vitamins, and supplements with the hope that my vision would return.

And this is my journey recovering my eyesight...

Side Note

Before I begin, I'd like to mention that I've had CRVO since September 2016. While I still experience occasional leaks, my vision has significantly improved, and the black spot is gone. Aside from a large floater, my eyesight is back to normal (20/25).

Recovering my vision required years of dedication, hard work, and perseverance. Reflecting on my journey, I believe that with the knowledge I have now, I could have healed my eye within a year or two of my diagnosis and avoided many of the complications that arose.

In this book, I briefly share my journey, the challenges I've faced, and the lessons I've learned. Additionally, I provide medical, scientific, and technical information about Central Retinal Vein Occlusion that I found on the web to offer answers and support to my fellow CRVO survivors.

I'd like to point out that you'll encounter dark sections like this one throughout the book. These sections are designed to separate my personal stories and treatment memories from the medical definitions. This approach aims to make the book less confusing, given the extensive technical information needed to explain the disease, its treatments, and its impact on CRVO patients. In these sections, I share my experiences, the processes I underwent, and insights I discovered online, in support groups, or from books. Please remember that my personal stories about healing my vision are not standard medical treatments or scientific conclusions but rather my own findings, theories, and revelations.

2

My Story

Central Retinal Vein Occlusion (CRVO) affects approximately 2.5 million people worldwide[1] and is one of the most common retinal vascular disorders after diabetic retinopathy. Over 85-90% of the cases occur in people over 55[2]. The chances of getting it increase with age, yet CRVO does occur in younger patients, though it is less common than in older adults.

Some studies suggest that around 10-15% of CRVO cases occur in people under the age of 40, and there is evidence to suggest that CRVO is more prevalent in men than in women, especially in older age groups. However, the gender difference in younger patients is not as well documented[4].

The most common causes of Retinal Vein Occlusion are high blood pressure, diabetes, glaucoma, and blood disorders. However, up to 30% of CRVO cases come from unknown causes[4], which is my situation.

When I was diagnosed with CRVO, I was in shock. How could this have happened to me? I didn't have any of the known causes like heart disease or diabetes, and the surprising part was that I never had eye issues before, so I didn't know what to do. At the time, I was in my early fifties and had been diagnosed with Hyperthyroidism. I had an adverse reaction to levothyroxine, which caused migraine headaches and severe tension in my eyes, but I had stopped taking the medication months before, so I couldn't tell if that was the culprit.

MY STORY

The night before my first leakage, it felt like I was having a bad allergy attack. My right eye was extremely itchy and was also twitching. I remember rubbing it very hard just before I fell asleep. When I woke early the following morning, it was like a scene from a horror movie. On the outside, my eye looked normal—no bruises, no blood, no signs of damage, but on the inside, my vision had an enormous black, bloody-looking spot, and I could barely see out of it.

I will admit I was very naive when it came to doctors or taking medication. I just never had to deal with it much until the thyroid issues. At first, I thought the eye condition was temporary, so I didn't panic. I calmly called my doctor and waited patiently to see the eye specialist, which didn't happen for two weeks. The first eye doctor they sent me wasn't an expert on my condition, and within minutes of seeing my test results, he sent me to an ophthalmologist. He didn't explain what he thought I had but stressed that it looked bad and that I needed to see the specialist right away.

At the time, I still wasn't freaking out. I remember thinking that I'd go to this expert doctor, and she'd give me some kind of medication—and then *POOF!* The large black spot would disappear, and my vision would be restored. However, that didn't happen. Instead, the specialist, a tiny lady with a high-pitched laugh, told me that I had an eye stroke and needed to get an injection. She didn't explain much of anything about my condition and then instructed her assistant to take photos of my eye. Moments later, she gave me the injection and told me to come back in four weeks.

To say I was confused is an understatement. I went home utterly frantic, and even though I could barely see, I turned on my computer and did a search for what an eye stroke was. The web pointed out that it was a condition called Retinal Vein Occlusion, and there were two types: Branch Retinal Vein Occlusion (BRVO) and the more severe type Central Retinal Vein Occlusion (CRVO). I remember praying to God, "Please don't let me have the bad one...," and then, much to my dismay, I was diagnosed with a severe case of Central Retinal Vein Occlusion.

Endnotes

[1] CRVO Informational Guide - angio.org. https://www.angio.org/downloads/Informational_Guide-Science_of_CRVO.pdf.

[2] Central Retinal Vein Occlusion - EyeWiki. https://eyewiki.aao.org/Central_Retinal_Vein_Occlusion.

[3] Diagnosis and Management of Central Retinal Vein Occlusion. https://www.aao.org/eyenet/article/diagnosis-of-central-retinal-vein-occlusion.

[4] The Causes and Treatment of Central Retinal Vein Occlusion: What Do We .... https://www.aao.org/education/current-insight/causes-treatment-of-central-retinal-vein-occlusion.

CENTRAL RETINAL VEIN OCCLUSION

3

What is CRVO?

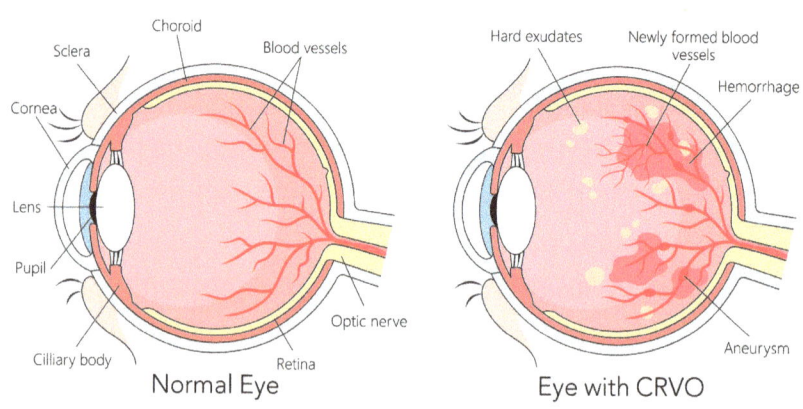

Normal Eye   Eye with CRVO

When the ophthalmologist told me that I had an eye stroke, she wasn't using the actual name for my condition. The technical term is Retinal Vein Occlusion, and in my case, it was Central Retinal Vein Occlusion, better known as CRVO. Sometimes, doctors refer to it as an eye stroke because it's easier for the patient to understand and comprehend what is happening to them[1].

There are two types of Retinal Vein Occlusions:

1. Central Retinal Vein Occlusion (CRVO)
2. Branch Retinal Vein Occlusion (BRVO)

Central Retinal Vein Occlusion happens when the primary vein responsible for draining blood from the light-sensitive layer at the back of your eye becomes obstructed. This blockage causes blood and fluid to leak into the retina, leading to swelling and vision problems[10]. It usually happens when a blood clot or when a larger blood vessel presses down on the vein[10]. When the vein is blocked, blood and fluid spill out into the retina. The macula, which is the part of the retina that is responsible for central vision, can swell from this fluid, affecting your vision[10].

Eventually, without blood circulation, the nerve cells in the eye can die, leading to further vision loss[10].

Branch Retinal Vein Occlusion occurs when one of the smaller veins in the retina gets blocked. This blockage causes blood and fluid to leak into the retina, leading to swelling and vision problems. It is considered less severe than CRVO. Its main symptoms include sudden blurry vision or vision loss in part of one eye. You might also see floaters, which are dark spots or lines in your vision. BRVO is often caused by conditions that affect blood flow, like high blood pressure, diabetes, or hardening of the arteries. It's more common in people over 50[13].

What are the technical differences between CRVO & BRVO?

CENTRAL RETINAL VEIN OCCLUSION (CRVO)

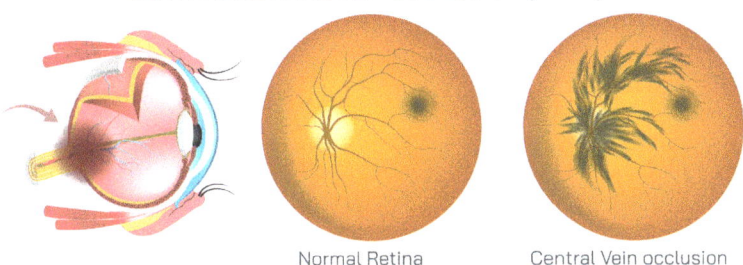

Normal Retina   Central Vein occlusion

CRVO's Key Points:

- Location: CRVO occurs in the retina's main vein.

- Vision Loss: It leads to sudden, profound, but painless vision loss in one eye. Most people with CRVO can barely count fingers or see light from the affected eye.

- Risk Factors: Commonly caused by a clot or embolus from the neck (carotid) artery or the heart. Underlying high blood pressure, carotid artery disease, cardiac valvular disease, or diabetes may contribute.

- Severity: Considered an "eye stroke."
- Diagnostic Work-Up: A comprehensive cardiovascular evaluation is recommended for all patients with CRVO[14].

BRVO's Key Points:

- Location: BRVO occurs in a smaller vein within the retina.
- Vision Loss: Typically results in localized vision loss in part of the visual field.
- Risk Factors: Associated with high blood pressure or high cholesterol.
- Prevalence: BRVO is six to seven times more common than CRVO.
- Treatment: Management focuses on underlying risk factors and may include laser therapy or anti-VEGF injections.

WHAT IS CRVO?

Both types of retinal vein occlusions can lead to complications such as macular edema, which is the swelling of the central part of the retina, and the growth of abnormal blood vessels, which can further impact vision[12]. The most common symptom of RVO is vision loss or blurry vision in part or all of one eye. It can happen suddenly or become worse over several hours or days. Sometimes, you can lose all vision suddenly. You may also notice floaters, dark spots, lines, or squiggles in your vision. These are shadows from tiny clumps of blood leaking into the vitreous from retinal vessels[10]. The main goal of treatment is to keep your vision stable. This is usually done by sealing off any leaking blood vessels in the retina, usually with anti-VEGF eye injections[10].

CRVO and BRVO are classified into two groups:

1. Non-ischemic (mild cases)
2. Ischemic (severe cases)

CRVO: Non-ischemic & Ischemic

1. Non-ischemic Central Retinal Vein Occlusion is a mild condition in which blood flow is reduced, resulting in leaky blood vessels in the retina[4]. It is considered the second most common retinal vascular disease in older adults after diabetic retinopathy[3][4]. It accounts for about 75% of cases of CRVO and is considered a less severe form with better visual outcomes for patients[5]. However, it is important to note that non-ischemic CRVO can develop into ischemic CRVO.

2. Ischemic CRVO is a more severe type of CRVO, a common retinal vascular disease[3][4]. In Ischemic CRVO, small retinal blood vessels are closed off[7][8]. Patients

with Ischemic CRVO often have worse vision with less chance for improvement[7][8]. One of the complications of this condition is that the eye may cause new blood vessels to grow, and these new vessels can clog the outflow of normal eye fluids[7][8]. This situation can further impact the vision of the patient.

BRVO: Non-ischemic & Ischemic

1. Non-ischemic Branch Retinal Vein Occlusion involves less severe blockage and reduced blood flow, leading to leaky blood vessels in the retina. It generally has a better prognosis and fewer complications[19][20].

2. Ischemic BRVO involves more severe blockage, significantly reducing blood flow and oxygen to the retina. It is defined by more than five-disc diameters of non-perfusion on fluorescein angiography (FA). Ischemic BRVO can lead to more serious complications, including the growth of abnormal blood vessels[19][20].

Typically, Retinal Vein Occlusions affect only one eye, and while some individuals may not experience any pain or symptoms, many people with CRVO or BRVO suffer from blurry vision. The good news is that early treatment can help reduce the risk of vision loss[5]. If ischemic RVO is suspected, it's important to consult a healthcare professional for diagnosis and treatment. They can provide appropriate guidance based on the individual's eye condition and health history.

Moving forward… now that I've defined the different types of Retinal Vein Occlusions, I will primarily focus on my condition, CRVO, for the remainder of the book to share my experiences with the disease. However, I will also include information on Branch Retinal Vein Occlusion when relevant or potentially helpful to the reader.

Endnotes

[1] Cleveland Clinic. Eye Stroke. https://my.clevelandclinic.org/health/diseases/24127-eye-stroke

[2] National Institute of Health (NIH). What is CRVO? https://www.nei.nih.gov/learn-about-eye-health/eye-conditions-and-diseases/central-retinal-vein-occlusion-crvo

[3] American Academy of Ophthalmology. EyeWiki. Central Retinal Vein Occlusion. https://eyewiki.aao.org/Central_Retinal_Vein_Occlusion

[4] All About Vision. Retinal vein occlusion (RVO): Causes, symptoms and treatments. https://www.allaboutvision.com/conditions/retina/retinal-vein-occlusion/

[5] Prevent Blindness. What is CRVO? https://preventblindness.org/central-retinal-vein-occlusion/

[6] Cleveland Clinic. Retina. https://my.clevelandclinic.org/health/body/22694-retina-eye

[7] American Society of Retina Specialists. The Foundation. Central Retinal Vein Occlusion. https://www.asrs.org/content/documents/fact-sheet-21-lp-central-retinal-vein-occlusion-2020_1_asrs.pdf

[8] Frontiers. Review: The Development of Risk Factors and Cytokines in Retinal Vein Occlusion. https://www.frontiersin.org/articles/10.3389/fmed.2022.910600/full

[9] National Institute of Health (NIH). Vision improvement is long-lasting with treatment for blinding blood vessel condition. https://www.nih.gov/news-events/news-releases/vision-improvement-long-lasting-treatment-blinding-blood-vessel-condition

[10] What Is Central Retinal Vein Occlusion (CRVO)?. https://www.aao.org/eye-health/diseases/what-is-central-retinal-vein-occlusion.

[11] Retinal Vein Occlusion: Causes, Types & Treatment - Cleveland Clinic. https://my.clevelandclinic.org/health/diseases/14206-retinal-vein-occlusion-rvo.

[12] What Is a Retinal Vein Occlusion? - American Academy of Ophthalmology. https://www.aao.org/eye-health/diseases/retinal-vein-occlusion-3.

[13] What Is Branch Retinal Vein Occlusion (BRVO)?. https://www.aao.org/eye-health/diseases/what-is-branch-retinal-vein-occlusion.

[14] Eye Strokes - Retinal Artery and Retinal Vein Occlusions - All About Vision. https://www.allaboutvision.com/conditions/eye-occlusions.htm.

[15] Branch Retinal Vein Occlusion - Patients - The American Society ... - ASRS. https://www.asrs.org/patients/retinal-diseases/24/branch-retinal-vein-occlusion.

[16] Retinal Vein Occlusion (BRVO and CRVO) - coloradoretina.com. https://www.coloradoretina.com/conditions/retinal-vein-occlusion-brvo-and-crvo.

[17] Retinal Vein Occlusion - College of Optometrists. https://www.college-optometrists.org/clinical-guidance/clinical-management-guidelines/retinal-vein-occlusion.

[18] Retinal Vein Occlusion - EyeWiki. https://eyewiki.aao.org/Retinal_Vein_Occlusion.

[19] Branch Retinal Vein Occlusion - EyeWiki. https://eyewiki.org/Branch_Retinal_Vein_Occlusion.

[20] Retinal Vein Occlusion (RVO) - Royal College of Ophthalmologists. https://www.rcophth.ac.uk/wp-content/uploads/2015/07/Retinal-Vein-Occlusion-Guidelines-Executive-Summary-2022.pdf.

4

The Symptoms

Central Retinal Vein Occlusion has many symptoms and they can vary, but the most common ones include:

- Vision loss or blurred vision: This can affect part or all of one eye and may happen suddenly or worsen over several hours or days[1][2].

- A big black or bloodish spot in your vision: This symptom is often related to the leakage of blood and fluid into the retina[4][5]. These spots are typically due to small blood clumps leaking from the retina and moving across the eye[4].

THE SYMPTOMS

- Eye floaters: These are dark spots, lines, or squiggles in your vision caused by tiny clumps of blood leaking into the retinal vessels' vitreous[1].

- Eye pain or pressure: This is more common in severe cases[2][3].

- Distorted vision: Seeing shapes as wavy or bent[3].

If you are experiencing any of these symptoms, it is essential to seek prompt medical attention immediately. Please DO NOT wait weeks for your general practitioner to schedule an appointment like I did. Contact your physician and ask to see an ophthalmologist or specialist right away. If they say you need approval from your insurance company, call them immediately. After all that, if you can't get an appointment, go to the emergency room so that they can perform the required tests, evaluate your symptoms, and stabilize your eye. Remember, every second that you wait could result in further vision loss.

Endnotes

[1] What Is Central Retinal Vein Occlusion (CRVO)? https://www.aao.org/eye-health/diseases/what-is-central-retinal-vein-occlusion.

[2] Central Retinal Vein Occlusion (CRVO) | National Eye Institute. https://www.nei.nih.gov/learn-about-eye-health/eye-conditions-and-diseases/central-retinal-vein-occlusion-crvo.

[3] Central Retinal Vein Occlusion: Symptoms, Causes, Treatment - Healthgrades. https://www.healthgrades.com/right-care/eye-health/central-retinal-vein-occlusion.

[4] Central retinal vein occlusion: Symptoms, causes, and more. https://www.medicalnewstoday.com/articles/central-retinal-vein-occlusion.

[5] Diagnosis and Management of Central Retinal Vein Occlusion. https://www.aao.org/eyenet/article/diagnosis-of-central-retinal-vein-occlusion.

5

What Causes it?

How does one get CRVO? Well, the exact cause of the disease is unclear, but Central Retinal Vein Occlusion is primarily caused by a blood clot or reduced blood flow in the central retinal vein, which is responsible for draining blood from the retina[1][2]. This blockage can cause pressure and fluid to build up, leading to swelling and damage to the inner eye[2].

There are a variety of factors that can raise the risk of one developing CRVO, such as:

- Diabetes [1][2]
- Glaucoma [1][2]

- Hardening of the arteries [1][2]
- High blood pressure [1][2]

As in my case, many patients do not know how they got the disease in the first place and feel helpless and lost because they do not know what lifestyle changes to make to prevent further damage or to stop the disease from causing a blockage in their good eye. Here are some factors that contribute to the disease:

- Age: Being over 50 years old [6].
- Smoking: This can damage blood vessels and increase the risk of blood clots [6].
- Ethnicity: Some studies suggest that being African American may increase the risk [6].
- Medications: Certain medications, including diuretics and oral contraceptives, can contribute to the risk [6].

- Compression of the retinal vein: This can occur when the retinal vein crosses paths with the retinal artery, especially if the artery is stiffened from aging or plaque buildup[5].

These factors, along with high blood pressure, diabetes, glaucoma, and arteriosclerosis, can all contribute to the development of CRVO[7][8].

How does CRVO damage the eyes?

After blood leaks into the eye, fluid collects in the macula, causing swelling and blurring central vision—this condition is known as macular edema. Common signs of macular edema following CRVO include vision loss (partial or complete), blurred vision, distorted vision, and faded colors[9].

The macula is responsible for sharp, detailed vision, which we need for activities like reading or driving. Fluid leakage from damaged blood vessels into the macula causes swelling and vision problems[9].

During this time, the retina may become deprived of oxygen (ischemia), leading to the growth of abnormal blood vessels. Some individuals with ischemic CRVO develop neovascular glaucoma, where these abnormal blood vessels increase eye pressure, causing pain and severe vision loss. Neovascular glaucoma can take three months or longer to develop after CRVO[9]. If you suffer from any of these symptoms, contact your doctor right away.

Endnotes

[1] Central Retinal Vein Occlusion (CRVO) | National Eye Institute. https://www.nei.nih.gov/learn-about-eye-health/eye-conditions-and-diseases/central-retinal-vein-occlusion-crvo.

[2] What Is Central Retinal Vein Occlusion (CRVO)?. https://www.aao.org/eye-health/diseases/what-is-central-retinal-vein-occlusion.

[3] Central Retinal Vein Occlusion - ASRS. https://www.asrs.org/content/documents/fact-sheet-21-central-retinal-vein-occlusion-2020_1_asrs.pdf.

[4] Central Retinal Vein Occlusion - Patients - The American Society of …. https://www.asrs.org/patients/retinal-diseases/22/central-retinal-vein-occlusion.

[5] Central Retinal Vein Occlusion: Symptoms, Causes, Treatment - Healthgrades. https://www.healthgrades.com/right-care/eye-health/central-retinal-vein-occlusion.

[6] The Causes and Treatment of Central Retinal Vein Occlusion: What Do We …. https://www.aao.org/education/current-insight/causes-treatment-of-central-retinal-vein-occlusion.

[7] Central retinal vein occlusion: Symptoms, causes, and more. https://www.medicalnewstoday.com/articles/central-retinal-vein-occlusion.

[8] Retinal Vein Occlusion: Causes, Types & Treatment - Cleveland Clinic. https://my.clevelandclinic.org/health/diseases/14206-retinal-vein-occlusion-rvo.

[9] Prevent Blindness. What is CRVO? https://www.preventblindness.org/central-retinal-vein-occlusion

6

Known Treatments

There aren't many options when it comes to treating CRVO or BRVO, and the available treatments are generally standard procedures. The main goal of treatments is to keep your eyes and vision stable. Most doctors focus on stopping abnormal blood vessels from growing and leaking in the retina to prevent swelling of the macula. Here are some of the most commonly performed treatments:

1. Anti-VEGF Injections

Roughly 65% of CRVO patients are treated with anti-VEGF drugs that help reduce the growth of abnormal blood vessels and decrease macular edema. Anti-VEGF (vascular endothelial growth factor) drugs are typically used in cancer treatment. These drugs work by inhibiting the growth of new blood vessels, a process known as angiogenesis, which is crucial for tumor growth and metastasis. By blocking VEGF, these drugs can help starve tumors of the blood supply they need to grow[9].

Due to their remarkable ability to prevent abnormal blood vessel growth, anti-VEGF drugs have become vision-saving treatments for patients with CRVO, BRVO, age-related macular degeneration, and diabetic macular edema[9].

Common anti-VEGF medications include:

- Avastin (Bevacizumab)
- Eylea (Aflibercept)
- Lucentis (Ranibizumab)

2. Steroid Injections

Steroid injections for the eye are used to treat various conditions that cause swelling or inflammation in the retina or other parts of the eye. These injections help reduce inflammation and fluid leakage, which can improve vision and prevent further damage[10][11].

a. Conditions treated with steroid injections:

- Macular edema (swelling in the central part of the retina)
- Diabetic macular edema (DME)
- Uveitis (inflammation of the middle layer of the eye)
- Retinal vein occlusion (blockage of veins in the retina)[10][11]

b. Commonly used steroid injections include:

- Triesence (triamcinolone acetonide) is a corticosteroid used to treat inflammation in various parts of the body, including the eye. It works by reducing inflammation and suppressing the immune response[12].

- Kenalog (triamcinolone acetonide) is also a corticosteroid used to treat various inflammatory conditions[10][11]. It works by reducing the body's immune response to decrease inflammation and alleviate symptoms like swelling[13].

3. Laser Treatment

Laser photocoagulation is a treatment used for certain cases of Central Retinal Vein Occlusion (CRVO), particularly when there is a risk of complications like neovascularization (abnormal blood vessel growth) or increased eye pressure. It involves using a laser to create tiny burns on the retina. This helps to reduce the risk of bleeding by sealing off leaking blood vessels and prevent neovascularization by reducing the oxygen demand of the retina, which can help prevent the growth of abnormal blood vessels[14][16].

Types of Laser Photocoagulation:

- Panretinal Photocoagulation (PRP): This is often used for severe CRVO cases. It involves making multiple laser burns across the retina to reduce the risk of neovascularization[14][16].

- Focal Laser Treatment: This targets specific areas of leakage or swelling in the retina.

It is important to note that Ischemic CRVO patients are more likely to require laser treatment due to the higher risk of neovascularization. Non-ischemic CRVO patients typically do not require laser treatment, as neovascularization is less common[15].

Benefits and Risks of Laser Treatment:

- Benefits: It can help prevent severe complications and preserve vision.

- Risks: Potential side effects include loss of peripheral vision, night vision issues, and possible damage to the retina if not done correctly[14][16].

4. Vitrectomy Surgery

In some cases, this surgery might be performed in the management of Central Retinal Vein Occlusion (CRVO), particularly when there are complications like vitreous hemorrhage that obstruct other treatments. Vitrectomy involves removing the vitreous gel from the eye. This is done using a vitrectomy probe, which cuts and removes the gel.

a. The procedure also allows the surgeon to:

- Clear any blood from the vitreous cavity.
- Remove scar tissue that may be pulling on the retina.
- Perform other necessary treatments like laser photocoagulation (PRP) if needed[15][16].

b. Vitrectomy is typically indicated for:

- Vitreous hemorrhage: When blood in the vitreous cavity prevents adequate laser treatment.
- Tractional retinal detachment: Caused by scar tissue pulling on the retina[3].

c. Benefits and Risks of Vitrectomy Surgery:

- Benefits: Can improve vision by clearing the vitreous cavity and allowing other treatments to be applied effectively.
- Risks: Potential complications include infection, bleeding, and retinal detachment[15][16].

5. Managing Underlying Conditions

Controlling underlying conditions such as high blood pressure, diabetes, and glaucoma is crucial for preventing and mitigating the effects of CRVO[2][4].

Here are some key steps:

a. Hypertension: High blood pressure is a significant risk factor for CRVO. Managing hypertension through:

- Medication: As prescribed by your doctor.
- Lifestyle changes: Such as reducing salt intake, regular exercise, and maintaining a healthy weight[3].

b. Manage Diabetes: Diabetes can damage blood vessels, increasing the risk of CRVO. Effective diabetes management includes:

- Monitoring blood sugar levels: Regularly checking and maintaining them within the target range.

- Diet and exercise: Following a balanced diet and staying active[3].

c. Cholesterol Levels: High cholesterol can contribute to vascular problems. Managing cholesterol involves:

- Medication: Statins or other cholesterol-lowering drugs as prescribed.
- Diet: Eating a heart-healthy diet low in saturated fats and trans fats[3].

d. Avoid Smoking: Smoking damages blood vessels and increases the risk of CRVO. Quitting smoking can significantly reduce this risk[17].

e. Regular Check-ups: Regular eye exams and check-ups with your healthcare provider can help monitor and manage these conditions effectively[3].

f. Healthy Lifestyle: Adopting a healthy lifestyle overall can help manage underlying conditions:

- Regular physical activity: At least 30 minutes of moderate exercise most days of the week.

- Healthy diet: Rich in fruits, vegetables, whole grains, and lean proteins.

- Weight management: Maintaining a healthy weight[17].

g. Medications: Taking medications as prescribed for any underlying conditions is essential. This includes antihypertensives, antidiabetics, and cholesterol-lowering drugs[3]. By effectively managing these underlying conditions, you can reduce the risk of CRVO and its complications.

6. Monitoring and Follow-Up

Monitoring and follow-up are crucial for managing Central Retinal Vein Occlusion (CRVO) to prevent complications and preserve vision. Here's a comprehensive plan:

a. Initial Assessment

Baseline Evaluation: Includes a detailed eye examination, fundus photography, fluorescein angiography, and optical coherence tomography (OCT) to assess the extent of retinal damage and macular edema[3][18].

b. Regular Follow-Up Visits

- Frequency: Monthly check-ups are recommended initially, especially for ischemic CRVO, to monitor for complications like neovascularization and macular edema[35].

- Examinations: Each visit should include visual acuity testing, intraocular pressure measurement, and a thorough retinal examination[3][18].

c. Monitoring for Complications

- Macular Edema: Regular OCT scans to detect and measure macular edema. Early detection allows timely treatment with anti-VEGF injections or steroids[3][18].

- Neovascularization: Regular fundus examinations and fluorescein angiography to monitor for abnormal blood vessel growth. Panretinal photocoagulation (PRP) may be needed if neovascularization is detected[18].

d. Managing Underlying Conditions

- Systemic Risk Factors: Regular monitoring and management of hypertension, diabetes, and hyperlipidemia. This includes routine blood pressure checks, blood sugar monitoring, and lipid profiles[3].

- Lifestyle Modifications: Encouraging a healthy lifestyle, including a balanced diet, regular exercise, and smoking cessation[3].

e. Long-Term Follow-Up

- Frequency: After the initial intensive monitoring period, follow-up visits can be spaced out to every 1-6 months, depending on the stability of the condition[5].

- Continued Monitoring: Ongoing assessment of visual function and retinal health to detect any late-onset complications[3].

f. Patient Education

- Symptoms Awareness: Educate patients about the symptoms of complications, such as sudden vision changes, and the importance of seeking immediate medical attention if they occur[3].

- Adherence to Treatment: Emphasize the importance of adhering to prescribed treatments and follow-up schedules[3].

By following this comprehensive monitoring and follow-up plan, patients with CRVO can better manage their condition and reduce the risk of severe vision loss.

Endnotes

[1] Central Retinal Vein Occlusion (CRVO) | National Eye Institute. https://www.nei.nih.gov/learn-about-eye-health/eye-conditions-and-diseases/central-retinal-vein-occlusion-crvo.

[2] Retinal Vein Occlusion: Causes, Types & Treatment - Cleveland Clinic. https://my.clevelandclinic.org/health/diseases/14206-retinal-vein-occlusion-rvo.

[3] Diagnosis and Management of Central Retinal Vein Occlusion. https://www.aao.org/eyenet/article/diagnosis-of-central-retinal-vein-occlusion.

[4] New Treatment Found to Reduce Vision Loss from Central Retinal Vein

https://medicalxpress.com/news/2009-09-treatment-vision-loss-central-retinal.pdf

[5] What Is Central Retinal Vein Occlusion (CRVO)?. https://www.aao.org/eye-health/diseases/what-is-central-retinal-vein-occlusion.

[6] New Treatment Found to Reduce Vision Loss from Central Retinal Vein …. https://www.nei.nih.gov/about/news-and-events/news/new-treatment-found-reduce-vision-loss-central-retinal-vein-occlusion.

[7] Five Years of Anti-VEGF for RVO Offers VA Gains. https://www.aao.org/eyenet/article/five-years-of-anti-vegf-for-rvo-offers-va-gains.

[8] How Long Does Avastin Work? - American Academy of Ophthalmology. https://www.aao.org/eye-health/ask-ophthalmologist-q/how-long-does-avastin-work.

[9] What are anti-VEGF drugs (VEGF inhibitors)?. https://www.drugs.com/medical-answers/anti-vegf-drugs-3570820/.

[10] Injections to Treat Eye Conditions | National Eye Institute. https://www.nei.nih.gov/learn-about-eye-health/eye-conditions-and-diseases/diabetic-retinopathy/injections-treat-eye-conditions.

[11] Eye Injections - American Academy of Ophthalmology. https://www.aao.org/eye-health/treatments/eye-injections.

[12] Triesence (Triamcinolone Acetonide Injectable Suspension): Side Effects …. https://www.rxlist.com/triesence-drug.htm.

[13] KENALOG-40 Vial - Uses, Side Effects, and More - WebMD. https://www.webmd.com/drugs/2/drug-9275/kenalog-injection/details.

[14] Treatments for Central Retinal Vein Occlusion - Retina Today. https://retinatoday.com/articles/2013-jan/treatments-for-central-retinal-vein-occlusion.

[15] Diagnosis and Management of Central Retinal Vein Occlusion. https://www.aao.org/eyenet/article/diagnosis-of-central-retinal-vein-occlusion.

[16] Retinal vein occlusion: Treatment - UpToDate. https://www.uptodate.com/contents/retinal-vein-occlusion-treatment.

[17] Understanding central retinal vein occlusion treatment and symptoms.. https://www.alliedacademies.org/articles/understanding-central-retinal-vein-occlusion-treatment-and-symptoms.pdf.

[18] Management of Retinal Vein Occlusion – Consensus Document. https://karger.com/oph/article/226/1/4/255193/Management-of-Retinal-Vein-Occlusion-Consensus.

[19] National Eye Institute](https://www.nei.nih.gov/learn-about-eye-health/eye-conditions-and-diseases/central-retinal-vein-occlusion-crvo)

[20] Cleveland Clinic](https://my.clevelandclinic.org/health/diseases/14206-retinal-vein-occlusion-rvo)

PROFESSIONAL CARE

7

The Doctor's Visit

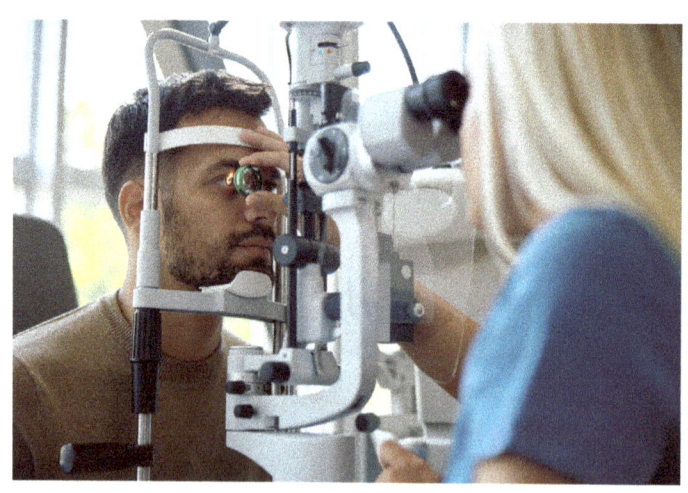

Patients with Central Retinal Vein Occlusion are typically treated by ophthalmologists, specifically retina specialists. These doctors specialize in diseases and conditions affecting the retina and vitreous of the eye. They are well-equipped to diagnose and manage CRVO, including administering treatments like anti-VEGF injections and steroid injections[4][5]. In some cases, patients may also need to see other specialists like an internist or a family doctor to manage underlying systemic conditions like diabetes or hypertension that can contribute to CRVO[3]. Hematologists may also treat patients if there is a need to investigate a suspected blood clotting disorder[3].

Here is a general outline of the various care and procedures that doctors or hospitals might perform when you need treatment for CRVO. I am lucky to have received my injections at one of the nation's best institutes for ophthalmology. It is a hospital setting, so my care will likely differ from yours (*note: I outline my appointment process at the end of this chapter).

Ophthalmologist Appointment:

When you visit a doctor for a CRVO (Central Retinal Vein Occlusion) appointment, here's what you can generally expect:

1. Medical History Review: The doctor will ask about your medical history, including any symptoms you're experiencing, your overall health, and any risk factors like diabetes, hypertension, or glaucoma.

2. Eye Examinations: A comprehensive eye exam will be conducted. This includes checking your visual acuity and examining the retina using tools like an ophthalmoscope or a slit lamp.

3. Diagnostic Tests:

- Optical Coherence Tomography (OCT): This imaging test provides detailed images of the retina, helping to identify any swelling or fluid accumulation.

- Fluorescein Angiography: A dye is injected into your arm, and pictures are taken as the dye travels through the blood vessels in your retina. This helps to identify any blockages or abnormal blood vessels.

- Blood Tests: These may be ordered to check for underlying conditions that could contribute to CRVO, such as blood clotting disorders[1][2].

- Fundus Photography: Images of the interior surface of the eye, including the retina, optic disc, macula, and posterior pole. In the context of Central Retinal Vein Occlusion (CRVO), fundus photos are used to document and monitor the condition of the retina. They can show issues like dilated and tortuous veins, swollen and twisted veins caused by blockage, optic disc edema, and macular edema [1][5].

4. Discussion of Findings: The doctor will explain the results of the tests and discuss the type of CRVO you have (ischemic or non-ischemic) and the severity of the condition.

5. Treatment Plan: Based on the findings, the doctor will recommend a treatment plan. This may include:

- Anti-VEGF Injections: These injections help reduce swelling and prevent the growth of abnormal blood vessels.
- Steroid Injections: These can help reduce inflammation and swelling in the retina.
- Laser Treatment: In some cases, laser therapy may be used to treat complications like neovascularization.

6. Follow-Up Appointments: Regular follow-up visits will be scheduled to monitor your condition and adjust the treatment plan as needed.

It's essential to ask any questions you have during the appointment to fully understand your condition and the proposed treatments. Then, make sure you set up your next appointment.

Endnotes

[1] Diagnosis and Management of Central Retinal Vein Occlusion. https://www.aao.org/eyenet/article/diagnosis-of-central-retinal-vein-occlusion.

[2] Central Retinal Vein Occlusion Central retinal vein occlusion, CRVO - ASRS. https://www.asrs.org/content/documents/fact-sheet-21-lp-central-retinal-vein-occlusion-2020_1_asrs.pdf.

[3] Central Retinal Vein Occlusion - Patients - The American Society of .... https://www.asrs.org/patients/retinal-diseases/22/central-retinal-vein-occlusion.

[4] Central Retinal Vein Occlusion (CRVO). https://www.nei.nih.gov/learn-about-eye-health/eye-conditions-and-diseases/central-retinal-vein-occlusion-crvo

[5] RVO Workup: When it's Necessary and What to Order. https://www.retina-specialist.com/article/rvo-workup-when-its-necessary-and-what-to-order

My Ophthalmology Visits

Step One: Medical History Review

An ophthalmic technician reviews my medical history, checks my eye pressure, and then performs a visual acuity test to see if my eyesight has changed since my last visit. Next, the technician uses eye drops to dilate my pupils and sends me to imaging.

Step Two: Fundus Photos

A technician takes pictures of the interior of my eye.

Step Three: Doctor's Examination

At this point, my ophthalmologist will review my data, examine my eye with a slit-lamp microscope, and then determine whether or not I need an injection.

Step Four: The Eye Injection

My ophthalmologist's assistant prepares for the injection by cleaning and numbing my eyes. This process usually takes 5 to 10 minutes. When she is done, she calls the doctor, prepares the medication, and places a speculum (a device to keep the eyelids open) in my eye.

Next, the doctor marks the injection spot, the assistant prepares a cotton swab, and the doctor gives the injection and then presses the swab to the site to prevent any leakage. Next, the nurse flushes my eye with drops and then checks my eye pressure, and if it's good, I can go.

8

Injections

Anti-VEGF Drugs

In 2004, anti-VEGF agents reached ophthalmic clinical practice, and since then, research into VEGF and potential inhibitors has continued, leading to the development of more effective anti-VEGF agents for CRVO patients[29].

Avastin typically lasts 4 to 8 weeks in the eye.

- Usage: Originally approved for cancer treatment, Avastin is used off-label for eye conditions like CRVO.

- **Mechanism:** It is an anti-VEGF (vascular endothelial growth factor) drug that reduces the growth of abnormal blood vessels and decreases fluid leakage in the eye.

- **Administration:** Given as an intravitreal injection (directly into the eye).

- **Cost:** As of July 2024, the cost of Avastin was around $849 for a supply of 4 milliliters[30].

- **Effectiveness:** Studies have shown that Avastin is as effective as Eylea in improving vision for CRVO patients[2].

Eylea lasts about 6 to 8 weeks in the eye.

- **Usage:** Approved specifically for eye conditions, including CRVO, diabetic macular edema, and wet age-related macular degeneration.

- **Mechanism:** Another anti-VEGF drug, Eylea, works by blocking VEGF and reducing swelling in the retina.

- Administration: Administered as an intravitreal injection, typically every 8 weeks after an initial series of monthly injections[1][2].

- Cost: As of July 2024, the cost of Eylea is approximately $1,800 to $2,000 per injection[31].

- Effectiveness: Clinical trials have demonstrated significant improvements in vision for patients with CRVO[1][2].

Lucentis typically lasts about 28 days in the eye, not 4 weeks.

- Usage: Specifically developed for eye conditions, including CRVO, diabetic macular edema, and wet age-related macular degeneration.

- Mechanism: Lucentis is an anti-VEGF drug that helps reduce macular edema and improve vision.

- Administration: it is usually given once a month, but after the initial injections, the schedule may change to once every 2-3 months, depending on the patient's response and the doctor's recommendation.[7].

- Cost: As of July 2024, it is similar to Eylea but more expensive than Avastin.
- Effectiveness: Extensively studied and shown to be effective in treating macular edema following CRVO[7].

While these anti-VEGF drugs are similar, they do not all work the same. Each anti-VEGF drug has its pluses and minuses, and you and your doctor must determine which drug best suits your condition.

Steroid Injections

Triesence lasts 3-4 months in the eye.

- Usage: it is used to reduce inflammation and swelling in the eye caused by conditions like CRVO. It helps manage macular edema, which is a common complication of CRVO[15].

- Mechanism: Triesence works by inhibiting the release of inflammatory substances in the body, but it doesn't specifically stabilize cell membranes or reduce capillary permeability[16].

- Administration: It is administered as an intravitreal injection, meaning it is injected directly into the vitreous humor of the eye. The typical dose is 4 mg (100 microliters of 40 mg/mL suspension), and the injection is performed under sterile conditions by a healthcare professional[17]. The procedure involves numbing the eye and monitoring for any adverse effects like increased intraocular pressure or infection[18].

- Cost: As of July 2024, the cost of Triesence can vary, but it is generally around $1,004 for a 1 mL vial of the 40 mg/mL suspension[19]. Prices may differ based on the pharmacy and location.

- Effectiveness: Triesence has been shown to be effective in reducing macular edema and improving visual acuity in patients with CRVO. Clinical studies have demonstrated significant improvements in vision and reduction in retinal thickness following treatment[20]. However, the effectiveness can vary among individuals, and some patients may require additional treatments.

Kenalog lasts for several weeks to a few months in the eye.

- Usage: it is used to reduce inflammation and swelling in the eye caused by CRVO. It helps manage macular edema, a common complication of CRVO[22].

- Mechanism: Kenalog works by decreasing the body's immune response and reducing inflammation. It inhibits the release of substances that cause inflammation and stabilizes cell membranes[23]. Specifically, it reduces the breakdown of the blood-retinal barrier and downregulates vascular endothelial growth factor (VEGF), which helps control macular edema[24].

- Administration: Kenalog is administered as an intravitreal injection, meaning it is injected directly into the vitreous humor of the eye. The typical dose for ocular conditions is 4 mg (100 microliters of 40 mg/mL suspension). The injection is performed under sterile conditions by a healthcare professional[4]. The procedure involves numbing the eye and monitoring for any adverse effects like increased intraocular pressure or infection[26].

- Cost: As of July 2024, the cost of Kenalog can vary, but it is generally around $19 for a 1 mL vial of the 40 mg/mL suspension[27]. Prices may differ based on the pharmacy and location.

- Effectiveness: Kenalog has been shown to be effective in reducing macular edema and improving visual acuity in patients with CRVO. Clinical studies have demonstrated significant improvements in vision and reduction in retinal thickness following treatment[28]. However, the effectiveness can vary among individuals, and some patients may require additional treatments.

Endnotes

[1] Avastin as effective as Eylea for treating central retinal vein occlusion. https://www.nih.gov/news-events/news-releases/avastin-effective-eylea-treating-central-retinal-vein-occlusion.

[2] Regeneron's Eylea Approved for Macular Edema Following CRVO. https://www.reviewofophthalmology.com/article/regenerons-eylea-approved-for-macular-edema-following-crvo.

[3] LUCENTIS® (ranibizumab) a Treatment Option for wAMD, DR & DME, mCNV, & RVO. https://bing.com/search?q=CRVO+drugs+Lucentis+details.

[4] Central Retinal Vein Occlusion - Patients - The American Society of .... https://www.asrs.org/patients/retinal-diseases/22/central-retinal-vein-occlusion.

[5] Avastin as effective as Eylea for treating central retinal vein occlusion. https://www.nei.nih.gov/about/news-and-events/news/avastin-effective-eylea-treating-central-retinal-vein-occlusion.

[6] Avastin as effective as Eylea for treating central retinal vein occlusion. https://medicalxpress.com/news/2017-05-avastin-effective-eylea-central-retinal.html.

[7] Treatment for RVO | LUCENTIS® (ranibizumab). https://www.lucentis.com/hcp/rvo.html.

[8] Central Retinal Vein Occlusion Central retinal vein occlusion, CRVO - ASRS. https://www.asrs.org/content/documents/fact-sheet-21-lp-central-retinal-vein-occlusion-2020_1_asrs.pdf.

[9] Clinical Trial Efficacy & Results for RVO - lucentis. https://www.lucentis.com/hcp/rvo/efficacy/clinical-trial-results.html.

[10] What is RVO? | LUCENTIS® (ranibizumab). https://www.lucentis.com/patient/rvo/about/what-is-rvo.html.

[11] LUCENTIS® (ranibizumab) a Treatment Option for wAMD, DR & DME, mCNV, & RVO. https://www.lucentis.com/.

[12] FDA approves Eylea for BRVO - American Academy of Ophthalmology. https://www.aao.org/education/headline/fda-approves-eylea-brvo.

[13] Your guide to EYLEA. https://www.sfda.gov.sa/sites/default/files/2022-11/CRVO%20patient%20brochure%20En.pdf.

[14] Your guide to EYLEA. https://www.medicines.org.uk/emc/rmm/619/Document.

[15] When to Use Steroids for Retinal Vein Occlusion - Retina Today. https://retinatoday.com/articles/2017-may-june/when-to-use-steroids-for-retinal-vein-occlusion.

[16] Triesence Injection: Uses, Dosage & Side Effects - Drugs.com. https://www.drugs.com/triesence.html.

[17] Untangling Retinal Vein Occlusion - American Academy of Ophthalmology. https://www.aao.org/eyenet/article/untangling-retinal-vein-occlusion.

[18] Evolving Role of Steroids in RVO and DME - retina-specialist.com. https://www.retina-specialist.com/article/evolving-role-of-steroids--in-rvo-and-dme.

[19] TRIESENCE suspension. TRIESENCE safely and effectively. See ... - Novartis. https://www.novartis.com/us-en/sites/novartis_us/files/triesence.pdf.

[20] TRIESENCE- triamcinolone acetonide injection, suspension - DailyMed. https://dailymed.nlm.nih.gov/dailymed/drugInfo.cfm?setid=3f045347-3e5e-4bbd-90f8-6c3100985ca5.

[21] Triamcinolone eye injection: Drug Basics and Frequently Asked ... - GoodRx. https://www.goodrx.com/triesence/what-is.

[22] Kenalog Injection: Uses, Side Effects, Interactions, Pictures ... - WebMD. https://www.webmd.com/drugs/2/drug-9275/kenalog-injection/details.

[23] Kenalog-40: Uses, Dosage, Side Effects, Warnings - Drugs.com. https://www.drugs.com/kenalog-40.html.

[24] Kenalog 10 Injection (Triamcinolone Acetonide Injectable … - RxList. https://www.rxlist.com/kenalog-10-injection-drug.htm.

[25] Triamcinolone Acetonide Injection: Uses, Side Effects … - WebMD. https://www.webmd.com/drugs/2/drug-9/triamcinolone-acetonide-injection/details.

[26] KENALOG -10 INJECTION (triamcinolone acetonide injectable suspension, USP). https://www.accessdata.fda.gov/drugsatfda_docs/label/2024/012041s051lbl.pdf.

[27] Kenalog-40 Dosage Guide - Drugs.com. https://www.drugs.com/dosage/kenalog-40.html.

[28] Kenalog-10 injection Uses, Side Effects & Warnings - Drugs.com. https://www.drugs.com/mtm/kenalog-10-injection.html.

[29] Anti-VEGF Therapy: Past, Present, and Future - Retina Today. https://retinatoday.com/articles/2021-may-june/anti-vegf-therapy-past-present-and-future.

[30] Avastin Prices, Coupons, Copay Cards & Patient Assistance. https://www.drugs.com/price-guide/avastin

[31] The Cost of Eylea Injection: What You Need to Know. https://eyesurgeryguide.org/the-cost-of-eylea-injection-what-you-need-to-know/

9

Laser Treatments

Laser photocoagulation is a treatment option for Central Retinal Vein Occlusion (CRVO). Here's a breakdown of its usage, mechanism, administration, cost, and effectiveness:

Usage: Laser photocoagulation is primarily used to treat complications of CRVO, such as neovascularization (abnormal blood vessel growth) and macular edema (swelling of the central retina). It is often considered when other treatments, like anti-VEGF injections, are not sufficient[3][4].

Mechanism: The treatment involves using a laser to create tiny burns on the retina. These burns help to seal leaking blood vessels, reduce swelling, and prevent the growth of new, abnormal blood vessels. This process helps to stabilize the retina and prevent further vision loss[3][4].

Administration: The procedure is typically performed in an ophthalmologist's office. The eye is numbed with anesthetic drops, and a special contact lens is placed on the eye to help focus the laser. The laser is then directed at the retina to create the necessary burns. The entire procedure usually takes about 15-30 minutes[3][4].

Cost: As of July 2024, the cost of laser photocoagulation can vary depending on the provider and location. On average, the procedure can cost around $1,390[8]. It's important to check with your insurance provider to see if the procedure is covered and what out-of-pocket expenses you might incur[10].

Effectiveness: Laser photocoagulation is effective in reducing the risk of complications like neovascularization and neovascular glaucoma. However, it is less effective in improving visual acuity. Studies have shown that while it can reduce macular edema, it does not significantly improve vision[4][11]. Therefore, it is often used in conjunction with other treatments like anti-VEGF injections for better overall outcomes[4].

Endnotes

[1] Central Retinal Vein Occlusion (CRVO) | National Eye Institute. https://www.nei.nih.gov/learn-about-eye-health/eye-conditions-and-diseases/central-retinal-vein-occlusion-crvo.

[2] Treatments for Central Retinal Vein Occlusion - Retina Today. https://retinatoday.com/articles/2013-jan/treatments-for-central-retinal-vein-occlusion.

[3] How Much Does a Photocoagulation Retinopathy Treatment Cost ... - MDsave. https://www.mdsave.com/procedures/photocoagulation-retinopathy-treatment/d580fdcc.

[4] Laser Photocoagulation: Uses, Benefits, Risks, Recovery-VerywellHealth.https://www.verywellhealth.com/laser-photocoagulation-5219365.

[5] Laser Photocoagulation in Retinal Vein Occlusion | Altintas .... http://www.ghrnet.org/index.php/IJOR/article/view/1623/2045.

[6] Retinal vein occlusion: Treatment - UpToDate. https://www.uptodate.com/contents/retinal-vein-occlusion-treatment.

[7] Diagnosis and Management of Central Retinal Vein Occlusion. https://www.aao.org/eyenet/article/diagnosis-of-central-retinal-vein-occlusion.

[8] Treatments for Central Retinal Vein Occlusion (CRVO). https://www.hey.nhs.uk/patient-leaflet/treatment-central-retinal-vein-occlusion-crvo/.

[9] Laser Therapy (Photocoagulation or Thermotherapy) for Retinoblastoma .... https://www.cancer.org/cancer/types/retinoblastoma/treating/laser-therapy.html.

[10] Retinal Vein Occlusion - American Academy of Ophthalmology. https://www.aao.org/education/munnerlyn-laser-surgery-center/retinal-vein-occlusion.

[11] Cost-effectiveness analysis of ranibizumab for retinal vein occlusion .... https://bmcophthalmol.biomedcentral.com/articles/10.1186/s12886-021-01997-1.

[12] Efficacy of panretinal laser in ischemic central retinal vein occlusion .... https://www.spandidos-publications.com/10.3892/etm.2018.7034.

[13] Evaluation and Management Of Retinal Vein Occlusion. https://www.reviewofophthalmology.com/article/evaluation-and-management-of-retinal-vein-occlusion.

[14] Clinical Guidelines - Royal College of Ophthalmologists. https://www.rcophth.ac.uk/wp-content/uploads/2015/07/Retinal-Vein-Occlusion-Guidelines-2022.pdf.

10

Vitrectomy Surgery

Vitrectomy surgery is one of the treatment options for Central Retinal Vein Occlusion (CRVO). Here's a detailed look at its usage, mechanism, administration, cost, and effectiveness:

Usage: Vitrectomy is typically used for CRVO when there is associated vitreous hemorrhage or persistent macular edema that does not respond to other treatments like anti-VEGF injections. It can also be considered in cases where there is significant traction on the retina[4].

Mechanism: The procedure involves removing the vitreous gel from the eye and may include peeling the internal limiting membrane (ILM). This helps to relieve traction on the retina and remove any blood or debris that might be causing vision problems. Additionally, it can help reduce the levels of cytokines, including vascular endothelial growth factor (VEGF), which contribute to macular edema[4][5].

Administration: Vitrectomy is performed under local or general anesthesia in an outpatient surgical center or hospital. The surgeon makes small incisions in the sclera (white part of the eye) to insert instruments that remove the vitreous gel. The procedure may also involve using a laser to repair the retina or injecting a gas bubble to keep the retina in place[3][5].

Cost: As of July 2024, the cost of vitrectomy surgery can vary widely depending on factors such as the surgeon, location, type of anesthesia, and whether insurance covers the procedure. On average, the cost ranges from $8,000 to $14,000 in the United States[9]. It's important to check with your insurance provider to understand your coverage and out-of-pocket expenses[8][10].

Effectiveness: Vitrectomy can be effective in reducing macular edema and improving visual acuity in some patients with CRVO. However, its effectiveness can vary, and it is not always the first-line treatment. Studies have shown mixed results, with some patients experiencing significant improvement in vision while others may not see substantial benefits[4][7]. It is often considered when other treatments have not been successful[4][12].

Endnotes

[1] Treatments for Central Retinal Vein Occlusion - Retina Today. https://retinatoday.com/articles/2013-jan/treatments-for-central-retinal-vein-occlusion.

[2] When to operate on RVO and when to (mostly) not. https://www.retina-specialist.com/article/when-to-operate-on-rvo-and-when-to-mostly-not

[3] Management of Retinal Vein Occlusion - Review of Ophthalmology. https://www.reviewofophthalmology.com/article/management-of-retinal-vein-occlusion.

[4] Central Retinal Vein Occlusion (CRVO) - Retina Center of NJ. https://www.retinacenternj.com/diseases-treatment/central-retinal-vein-occlusion-crvo.

[5] Vitrectomy Surgery: Use Cases, Procedure, Recovery, and Costs. https://www.visioncenter.org/surgery/vitrectomy/.

[6] Guide to Vitrectomy: Costs, Timelines & More - NVISION Eye Centers. https://www.nvisioncenters.com/eye-surgery/vitrectomy/.

[7] The Cost Of Vitrectomy - The Pricer. https://www.thepricer.org/the-cost-of-vitrectomy/.

[8] Vitrectomy and radial optic neurotomy for central retinal vein .... https://link.springer.com/article/10.1007/s00417-004-1046-0.

[9] Diagnosis and Management of Central Retinal Vein Occlusion. https://www.aao.org/eyenet/article/diagnosis-of-central-retinal-vein-occlusion.

[10] Surgery for Retinal Venous Occlusions - Review of Ophthalmology. https://www.reviewofophthalmology.com/article/surgery-for-retinal-venous-occlusions.

[11] When to Operate on RVO and When to (Mostly). Not https://dukeeyecenter.duke.edu/news/when-operate-rvo-and-when-mostly-not

[12] Treatment for retinal vein occlusion yields long-lasting vision gains .... https://www.news-medical.net/news/20220421/Treatment-for-retinal-vein-occlusion-yields-long-lasting-vision-gains-study-shows.aspx.

[13] en.wikipedia.org. https://en.wikipedia.org/wiki/Vitrectomy.

11

Complications

Anti-VEGF

CRVO injections, such as those for Avastin, Eylea, and Lucentis, can be very effective but do come with some potential complications. Here are some typical ones:

Common Anti-VEGF Complications:

- **Increased Intraocular Pressure:** This can occur shortly after the injection and usually resolves on its own.

- **Cataract Formation:** Repeated injections may increase the risk of developing cataracts over time.

COMPLICATIONS

- **Retinal Detachment:** Though rare, this is a serious complication where the retina detaches from the back of the eye[3], and it requires immediate attention.

- **Intraocular Hemorrhage:** Bleeding inside the eye can occur, which may affect vision[3].

- **White Out:** A "white out" typically describes a sudden loss of vision where everything appears white or very bright. This can be caused by various factors, including high eye pressure, retinal detachment, severe migraines, or other acute eye conditions[6].

- **Posterior Vitreous Detachment (PVD):** this occurs when the vitreous, a gel-like substance filling the eye, separates from the retina, causing floaters and flashes (tiny specks or cobwebs in your vision) of light[18][19]. PVD is a common age-related condition, and while it can occur after intravitreal injections, the exact incidence rates may vary.

Infectious Complications:

- Endophthalmitis: The incidence rate of infectious endophthalmitis varies with CRVO patients, but it's generally around 0.08% to 0.68% following intraocular procedures, not exactly 1 in 1000 patients[5].

- Sterile Endophthalmitis: This condition involves inflammation without infection, often presenting with acute and painless vision loss, dense vitreous opacity, and mild to moderate anterior segment reaction[3].

Other Complications:

- **Vitreous Hemorrhage:** Bleeding into the vitreous gel inside the eye, which can cause floaters or vision loss[4].

- **Neovascularization:** The growth of new, abnormal blood vessels can lead to complications like neovascular glaucoma[4].

Recurrence of Macular Edema:

- In between injections, there is a chance your eye will leak blood. This fluid accumulates in your macula, the central part of the retina responsible for sharp, detailed vision, and causes swelling, which can distort your vision, make things look blurry, and make colors appear washed out[7][8].

- Repeated Injections: these are often necessary as retinal edema can recur, requiring ongoing treatments[3].

Steroid Injection Complications

Steroid injections for treating Central Retinal Vein Occlusion (CRVO) can be effective, but they do come with potential complications. Here are some of the main ones:

1. Increased Intraocular Pressure: Steroid injections can cause a rise in the pressure inside the eye, which may lead to glaucoma if not managed properly[13].

2. Cataract Formation: Prolonged use of steroids can accelerate the development of cataracts, leading to clouding of the lens and vision impairment[13].

3. Infections: Though rare, there is a risk of infection at the injection site[12].

4. Retinal Detachment: This is a serious condition where the retina detaches from the back of the eye, potentially leading to vision loss[11].

5. Intraocular Hemorrhage: Bleeding inside the eye can occur, which may require additional treatment[11].

6. Sterile or Pseudo-Endophthalmitis: This is an inflammatory response that can mimic an infection but is not caused by bacteria[11].

It's important to discuss these potential risks with each of these injection types with your eye care specialist or doctor to understand how they might apply to your situation and ensure you receive the best possible care. Regular monitoring and follow-up appointments are crucial to manage any side effects promptly. If you notice any change in your vision or witness any of these issues, contact your doctor or ophthalmologist immediately.

Laser Treatment Complications

Laser photocoagulation is a common treatment for Central Retinal Vein Occlusion, but it can come with some complications. Here are a few potential issues:

1. Scotoma: This is a partial loss of vision or a blind spot in an otherwise normal visual field, which can occur if the heat from the laser affects the photoreceptors[13].

2. Foveal Burns: Inadvertent burns to the fovea can cause significant central vision loss[13].

3. Vitreous Hemorrhage: Bleeding into the vitreous humor of the eye can occur[14].

4. Retinal Detachment: When the retina pulls away from the back of the eye, it becomes a critical situation that requires immediate medical attention[14].

5. Neovascularization: Abnormal blood vessel growth can happen at the laser site[15].

6. Elevated Intraocular Pressure: This can lead to glaucoma if not managed properly[14].

While these complications can be serious, laser photocoagulation remains an important treatment option for managing CRVO. It's crucial to discuss these potential risks with your doctor beforehand.

Vitrectomy Surgery Complications

Vitrectomy surgery can be effective for CRVO, but like any surgical procedure, it comes with potential complications. Here are some possible issues:

1. Infection: There's a risk of developing an infection inside the eye, known as endophthalmitis[16].

2. Hemorrhaging: Bleeding can occur inside the eye during or after surgery[16].

3. Retinal Detachment: When the retina separates from the back of the eye, it leads to a critical condition requiring immediate medical intervention[16].

4. Cataract Formation: Vitrectomy Surgery can lead to the development of new cataracts or accelerate the progression of existing ones[16].

5. Increased or Decreased Eye Pressure: This can lead to glaucoma or hypotony (abnormally low eye pressure)

6. Inflammation: Redness, swelling, and pain can occur as a result of the surgery[17].

7. Need for Additional Surgery: Sometimes, further corrective surgeries may be necessary[16].

Even though these potential complications might be alarming, vitrectomy stands as a crucial and effective solution for managing severe cases of CRVO. Always ensure you discuss the risks and benefits with your ophthalmologist to make the best choice for your eye health.

Endnotes

[1] Evaluation and Management Of Retinal Vein Occlusion. https://www.reviewofophthalmology.com/article/evaluation-and-management-of-retinal-vein-occlusion.

[2] Treatments for Central Retinal Vein Occlusion (CRVO). https://www.hey.nhs.uk/patient-leaflet/treatment-central-retinal-vein-occlusion-crvo/.

[3] CRVO Informational Guide - Angio. http://www.angio.org/downloads/Informational_Guide-Science_of_CRVO.pdf.

[4] Central Retinal Vein Occlusion (CRVO) | National Eye Institute. https://www.nei.nih.gov/learn-about-eye-health/eye-conditions-and-diseases/central-retinal-vein-occlusion-crvo.

[5] Central Retinal Vein Occlusion - Patients - The American Society of .... https://www.asrs.org/patients/retinal-diseases/22/central-retinal-vein-occlusion.

[6] Ocular Hypertension vs Glaucoma: Are They The Same?. https://www.goodrxmedicine.com/blog/eyecare/ocular-hypertension-vs-glaucoma/.

[7] What Is Macular Edema? - American Academy of Ophthalmology. https://www.aao.org/eye-health/diseases/what-is-macular-edema.

[8] Macular Edema: Symptoms, Causes, Diagnosis, and Treatment - Healthline. https://www.healthline.com/health/eye-health/macular-edema.

[9] Central Retinal Vein Occlusion. https://eyewiki.org/Central_Retinal_Vein_Occlusion

[10] Cortisone Shots (Steroid Injections): Benefits & Side Effects. https://my.clevelandclinic.org/health/treatments/cortisone-shots-steroid-injections.

[11] Retinal Vein Occlusion: Causes, Types & Treatment - Cleveland Clinic. https://my.clevelandclinic.org/health/diseases/14206-retinal-vein-occlusion-rvo.

[12] When to Use Steroids for Retinal Vein Occlusion - Retina Today. https://retinatoday.com/articles/2017-may-june/when-to-use-steroids-for-retinal-vein-occlusion.

[13] Retinal Vein Occlusion - American Academy of Ophthalmology. https://www.aao.org/education/munnerlyn-laser-surgery-center/retinal-vein-occlusion.

[14] Guidelines for the Management of Retinal Vein Occlusion. https://www.retinsight.com/media/Guideline-1_2019_Schmidt-Erfurth-et-al_Ophtalmologica-242.pdf

[15] Surgery for Retinal Venous Occlusions - Review of Ophthalmology. https://www.reviewofophthalmology.com/article/surgery-for-retinal-venous-occlusions.

[16] Diagnosis and Management of Central Retinal Vein Occlusion. https://www.aao.org/eyenet/article/diagnosis-of-central-retinal-vein-occlusion.

[17] What Is a Posterior Vitreous Detachment? - American Academy of .... https://www.aao.org/eye-health/diseases/what-is-posterior-vitreous-detachment.

[18] Posterior Vitreous Detachment: Causes, Symptoms & Treatments. https://my.clevelandclinic.org/health/diseases/14413-posterior-vitreous-detachment.

COMPLICATIONS

[19] FDA: FDA warns consumers not to purchase or use certain eye drops from several major brands due to risk of eye infection. https://www.fda.gov/drugs/drug-safety-and-availability/fda-warns-consumers-not-purchase-or-use-certain-eye-drops-several-major-brands-due-risk-eye#:~:text=Walmart%20is%20removing%20the%20product,partial%20vision%20loss%20or%20blindness.

[20] Glaucoma and the Optic Nerve: Cupping and Progressive Effects - Healthline. https://www.healthline.com/health/eye-health/glaucoma-optic-nerve.

[21] Glaucoma and Eye Pressure | National Eye Institute. https://www.nei.nih.gov/learn-about-eye-health/eye-conditions-and-diseases/glaucoma/glaucoma-and-eye-pressure.

[22] YO Need to Know: Acute Angle Closure - American Academy of …. https://www.aao.org/young-ophthalmologists/yo-info/article/yo-need-to-know-acute-angle-closure.

[23] NIH. Posterior vitreous detachment following intravitreal drug injection. https://www.ncbi.nlm.nih.gov/pmc/articles/PMC3682090/

My CRVO Complications

Thankfully, I haven't had too many complications, but some of the ones that I have had were scary, painful, and really messed with my vision. Here is the list:

1) Posterior Vitreous Detachment (PVD) with a Weiss ring: Early on in my recovery, just a couple of hours after an injection, I had an enormous floater appear in my CRVO eye. It looked like a giant bug with wings and darted back and forth as my eye moved. It was called a Weiss ring floater, a more severe type of PVD, and it distorted my vision for years because of the way it separated from the retina. My vision became pinched in the center and elongated in height, similar to a funhouse mirror. Thankfully, after years of eye exercises and time, it's back to normal.

2) White Outs: For the last year, my vision in the CRVO eye has gone completely white immediately after an injection. It scares the heck out of me. The whiteout happens because my optic nerve is being compressed by extremely high intraocular eye pressure[21][22]. Thankfully, my nurse has had a few patients with the same issue and calmly massages my eye with very light pressure until I can see again. She had explained to me that the reason it was happening was because my eye was healthier and not as bloated as when I was leaking a lot of blood. She also mentioned that with some of her glaucoma patients, the doctor has to tap the eye to release the pressure. "Tapping the eye" is a medical procedure in which a small amount of fluid is drained from the eye to quickly reduce intraocular pressure (IOP) [23].

3) Corneal Abrasion: After a recent injection, hours later, when the numbing agent faded, I had a sharp stabbing pain in my eye. It was excruciating. I took two Advil, but the pain didn't go away. I called my doctor, but his office never returned my call, so I stayed in bed, waiting for the pain to subside, but it never did. Then, at midnight, when I couldn't take it anymore, I searched the web and learned that the eye speculum must have scratched the surface of my cornea. Luckily, I found a YouTube video that explained that I needed to lubricate the eye and put a bandage on it so that it would stop the eye from moving. Barely able to see, I drove up the block to the nearest CVS and bought Systane Nighttime Lubricant Eye Ointment (a gel lubricant), large gauze pads, and medical tape. By morning, the pain had subsided.

COMPLICATIONS

4) Cataracts: The repeated injections have accelerated the formation of cataracts in my CRVO eye. I was combating them with Can-C drops that worked great, but the FDA took them off the market in 2023, along with 26 other eyedrops, due to the potential risk of eye infections that could result in partial vision loss or blindness[20]. Luckily, they aren't too bad now.

5) Minor Issues: Other things like floaters, squigglies, darting black spots, and dry eyes, but thankfully all were manageable and painless.

12

After the Injection

Patients may experience some discomfort after receiving an injection for either CRVO or BRVO. Here are some things that you can expect:

1. Irritation and Scratchiness: It's common for the eye to feel irritated and scratchy for about a day after the injection[3]. Use lubricant eye drops like Systane Ultra Lubricant Eye Drops to moisten and lubricate and help manage symptoms of dry eye and ocular surface irritation.

2. Ocular Surface Irritation: This can last longer, especially if there's corneal epithelial breakdown or dryness induced by antiseptics used during the procedure[4].

3. Mild Pain or Redness: Some patients may experience mild pain or redness in the eye[5].

4. Blurred Vision: Temporary blurred vision can occur, but it usually resolves within a short period[5].

5. Floaters or Bloody Eye: Many times after the injection, a black spot will appear. These types of spots usually go away after a few hours. Also, sometimes tiny capillaries can break and cause the eye to have a bloody spot. It is not painful and usually goes away within a week or so.

What NOT to do after an eye injection

- **Avoid Rubbing Your Eye:** This can cause irritation or even infection.

- **No Heavy Lifting or Strenuous Activities:** These can increase eye pressure and potentially cause complications.

- **Avoid Swimming:** Pools and hot tubs can introduce bacteria to the eye.

- **Skip Eye Makeup:** For at least a day or two to prevent any potential irritation or infection.

- **Do Not Miss Follow-Up Appointments:** It's crucial to monitor your eye's healing process.

Endnotes

[1] Central Vein Occlusion - Retinal Consultants Medical Group. https://www.retinalmd.com/retina-conditions/central-vein-occlusion.

[2] Distinguishing Infection Post-Intravitreal Injection. https://www.reviewofophthalmology.com/article/distinguishing-infection-post-intravitreal-injection-41670.

[3] Instructions After Intravitreal Injections | Houston Retina Associates .... https://www.hretina.com/patient-resources/retinal-conditions/instructions-after-intravitreal-injections.

[4] Central Retinal Vein Occlusion (CRVO) | National Eye Institute. https://www.nei.nih.gov/learn-about-eye-health/eye-conditions-and-diseases/central-retinal-vein-occlusion-crvo.

[5] Central Retinal Vein Occlusion - Patients - The American Society of .... https://www.asrs.org/patients/retinal-diseases/22/central-retinal-vein-occlusion.

My CRVO Injection Experience

I'm not going to sugarcoat it—the idea of getting an injection in the eye is utterly terrifying. At first, I wanted nothing to do with them. I dreaded each appointment with a passion. But as time went on, about a year or so later, a realization dawned on me that these injections were the key to preserving my vision and maintaining a normal life. They became less of a nightmare and more of a lifeline.

In the early days, when my CRVO was at its worst and my eye was a tangle of engorged abnormal blood vessels, the pain after an injection was relentless. My eye would throb for days, leaving me bedridden and unable to do much of anything.

These days, the discomfort in my CRVO eye is minimal, and I find that I no longer need to rest after an injection. I can go about my day within a couple of hours of the treatment.

Interestingly, now that the engorged blood vessels have subsided, the aching pain has vanished. Occasionally, when my eye does leak, there is a mild ache, but it's nothing compared to the intense pain I experienced when I was first diagnosed.

13

Follow-up Appointments

A follow-up appointment after CRVO injections typically involves several key steps to monitor your eye's response to the treatment and ensure there are no complications:

1. Visual Acuity Test: This checks how well you can see and if there's been any improvement or decline in your vision.

2. Eye Examination: The doctor will examine your eye, often using a slit lamp, to look for any signs of inflammation, infection, or other issues.

3. Optical Coherence Tomography (OCT) or Fundus photos: This imaging test provides detailed pictures of the retina, helping the doctor assess the extent of macular edema (swelling) and other changes[1].

4. Intraocular Pressure Measurement: Checking the pressure inside your eye is important, especially if you have glaucoma or are at risk for it[2].

5. Discussion of Symptoms: Inform your ophthalmologist of any changes in your eyesight, symptoms, or side effects you've experienced since your last injection, such as pain, redness, or changes in vision[3].

Follow-up appointments are crucial for adjusting your treatment plan as needed and ensuring the best possible outcome for your vision. I do not recommend skipping them because every time you leak blood and the macula becomes swollen, it sets your progress back weeks or months. Don't risk it!

Endnotes

[1] Diagnosis and Management of Central Retinal Vein Occlusion. https://www.aao.org/eyenet/article/diagnosis-of-central-retinal-vein-occlusion.

[2] Untangling Retinal Vein Occlusion - American Academy of Ophthalmology. https://www.aao.org/eyenet/article/untangling-retinal-vein-occlusion.

[3] Retinal vein occlusion: Treatment - UpToDate. https://www.uptodate.com/contents/retinal-vein-occlusion-treatment.

[4] Evaluation and Management Of Retinal Vein Occlusion. https://www.reviewofophthalmology.com/article/evaluation-and-management-of-retinal-vein-occlusion.

[5] Central Vein Occlusion - Retinal Consultants Medical Group. https://www.retinalmd.com/retina-conditions/central-vein-occlusion.

HEALING THE EYE

14

Is CRVO Curable?

As of the fall of 2024, if you conducted a search of all the top medical and eye specialist websites around the world, you would get the same answer—no, CRVO is not curable. Then, the site would list all the standard treatments for the disease.

Unfortunately, CRVO does not have a high cure rate, and the prognosis varies from person to person. Mild cases may improve without treatment, but I wouldn't take a chance, so get the injection. Early intervention is crucial to maintaining vision and minimizing vision loss.

Can You Improve Your CRVO Condition?

Well, if you scour the internet for natural remedies to heal CRVO, you'd come up empty-handed. It seems the industry is solely focused on promoting conventional treatments for the condition. I've even had my first ophthalmologist laugh at me when I asked her if there were any diet changes that I could make to improve my condition, and she just cackled in that high-pitched voice of hers and said, "Do you think eating carrots is going to cure you?"

I had a hunch she was one of those doctors who dismissed the idea that foods and nutrients could have healing powers. Her reaction struck me as strange, given that many leading causes of CRVO typically stem from a patient's health or lifestyle choices. Thankfully, she was wrong—otherwise, I might still be blind. The truth is that many eye doctors and ophthalmologists are not there to cure the disease. The mysteries of how you got CRVO matter little to them. All they are concerned with is stopping the leakage and maintaining your vision. However, we CRVO survivors want to heal, and thus, there is so much to know.

The eyes are extraordinary because they offer a transparent window into our blood vessels, nerves, and connective tissues, revealing a wealth of health information. Conditions such as diabetes, high blood pressure, high cholesterol, heart disease, autoimmune disorders, and even brain tumors often manifest clues that can be detected in the eyes. These ailments are the primary culprits behind retinal vein occlusions.

Many people are unaware that an annual eye exam can catch these issues early on. The saying, "the eyes are the window to the soul," could easily be rephrased as, "the eyes are the window to our health," because when an eye doctor peers into them, they can spot if anything is out of the ordinary.

So, is CRVO curable?

Technically, there's no magical pill or treatment that will cure the disease. However, when you break CRVO down into three main components and treat them individually... **yes, I do believe it is possible to heal and regain your vision.**

So let's begin...

15

Exploring the Eye

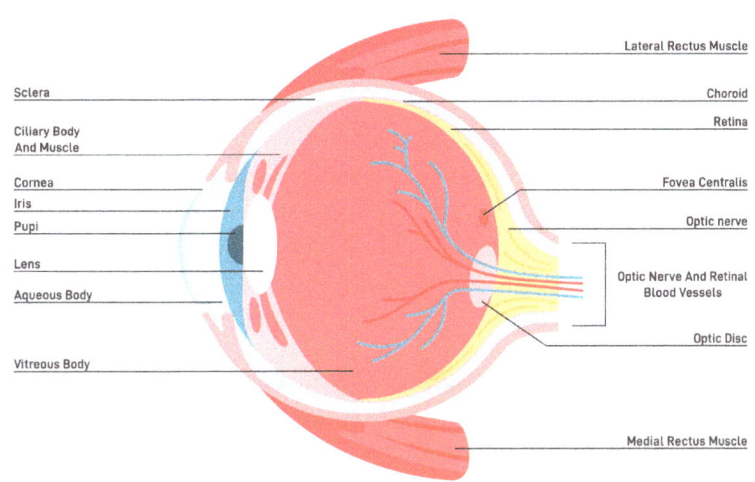

Eye Anatomy

The human eye is a complex and fascinating organ responsible for vision. It allows us to see by capturing light and converting it into electrical signals the brain can interpret as images. It is truly amazing, but what makes it even more remarkable is that some parts of the eye can actually heal themselves, and other parts have the ability to regenerate cells over time. In this chapter, I will explore the various components of the eye and their respective capacities for healing and explain why sometimes the eye does not heal itself.

Overview of the Eye's Major & Minor Components

1. Major Parts of the Eye include:

A) Cornea: The clear, dome-shaped surface that covers the front of the eye. It helps focus incoming light.

B) Iris: The colored part of the eye that controls the size of the pupil and, consequently, the amount of light that enters the eye.

C) Pupil: The black circular opening in the center of the iris that allows light to enter the eye.

D) Lens: Located behind the iris, it further focuses light onto the retina.

E) Retina: The light-sensitive layer at the back of the eye that contains photoreceptor cells (rods and cones). It converts light into electrical signals.

F) Optic Nerve: Transmits visual information from the retina to the brain.

2. Minor Parts of the Eye include:

A) Conjunctiva: A thin, clear membrane that covers the white of the eye and the inside of the eyelids. It keeps the eye moist by making mucus and tears[1].

B) Sclera: The white outer layer of the eyeball that provides structure and protection[2].

C) Aqueous Humor: A clear fluid in the front part of the eye (anterior chamber) that maintains eye pressure and nourishes the cornea and lens[1].

D) Vitreous Humor: A gel-like substance that fills the space between the lens and the retina, playing a crucial role in maintaining the eye's shape.[3].

E) Ciliary Body: Contains the ciliary muscle, which adjusts the lens for focusing and produces the fluid in the eye[3].

F) Choroid: A layer of blood vessels between the retina and the sclera that provides oxygen and nutrients to the eye[3].

G) Macula: A small, central area of the retina responsible for sharp, detailed central vision[4].

H) Fovea: The central part of the macula that provides the clearest vision of all[3].

These parts work together to capture light and convert it into images, allowing us to see the world around us[3].

Healing & Regenerating Abilities

Knowing which parts of the eye can heal or regenerate is essential for assessing potential vision recovery. For example, the cornea has a good regenerative capacity, while the retina and optic nerve have very limited ability to regenerate[8][9][10]. This knowledge helps in developing appropriate treatment plans and setting realistic expectations for vision restoration.

- **Cornea:** The cornea has a good ability to heal itself, especially the outer layer (epithelium). It can regenerate quickly from minor injuries[5].

- **Pupil:** The pupil itself is an opening and does not have regenerative capabilities. However, the muscles controlling the pupil, such as the iris muscles, can recover from minor injuries[6].

- **Lens:** The lens has limited regenerative capabilities. Lens epithelial cells can regenerate to some extent, but this ability declines with age[6].

- **Retina:** The retina has very limited regenerative capacity. So, the damage to the retina, especially the photoreceptors, is often permanent[6].

- **Optic Nerve:** The optic nerve does not regenerate naturally. Damage to the optic nerve typically results in permanent vision loss[7].

- **Conjunctiva:** The conjunctiva can heal from minor injuries and regenerate its epithelial cells[5].

- **Sclera:** The sclera has limited regenerative capabilities but can heal from minor injuries[6].

- **Aqueous Humor:** The aqueous humor is a fluid and does not regenerate, but it is continuously produced and drained by the eye[6].

- **Vitreous Humor:** The vitreous humor is a gel-like substance that does not regenerate. It remains largely unchanged throughout life[6].
- **Ciliary Body:** The ciliary body has limited regenerative capabilities but can recover from minor injuries[6].
- **Choroid:** The choroid has limited regenerative capabilities but can heal from minor injuries[6].
- **Macula:** The macula, part of the retina, has very limited regenerative capacity. Damage to the macula often results in permanent vision loss[6].
- **Fovea:** The fovea, located in the center of the macula, also has very limited regenerative capacity. Damage here can lead to significant vision loss[6].

Truthfully, it's not necessary to know all the components of the eye to aid its healing. However, I've provided this information to help you gain a better understanding of how it all works together.

Why the Eye Doesn't Heal Itself

As remarkable as the eye is, sometimes it doesn't know that it is injured due to a phenomenon known as immune privilege. This unique status limits the eye's inflammatory immune response to protect vision from being harmed by swelling and other tissue changes[15]. Essentially, the eye is designed to prevent an immune system overreaction that could damage sensitive visual tissues and impair vision. Because of this, immune privilege can sometimes prevent the eye from recognizing when it's being damaged. For example, severe eye conditions like glaucoma or retinal detachment often do not cause pain or immediate symptoms, making them harder to detect without regular eye examinations[14].

However, the body has mechanisms to respond to damage and stress. In the case of when Central Retinal Vein Occlusion (CRVO) occurs, several processes are triggered:

- **Inflammatory Response:** The body releases inflammatory mediators to address the damage[11][12].

- **Vascular Changes:** The blockage in the vein can lead to the release of vascular endothelial growth factor (VEGF), which promotes the growth of new blood vessels[11][12].

- **Edema:** Swelling in the retina, known as macular edema, can occur due to fluid leakage[11][12].

- **Neovascularization:** In severe cases, new, abnormal blood vessels may form, which can lead to further complications[13].

Summary

In conclusion, while immune privilege prevents the CRVO eye from recognizing that it is hurt, the body's immune system senses something is wrong and attempts to fix it by growing abnormal blood vessels to provide the eye with much-needed oxygen. Unfortunately, this well-intentioned repair can cause more harm. Yet, as vision worsens, it serves as a signal for the patient to seek an eye exam, which becomes the crucial first step in addressing the condition.

Endnotes

[1] Eye Anatomy: Parts of the Eye and How We See. https://www.aao.org/eye-health/anatomy/parts-of-eye.

[2] Eye Anatomy: Parts of the Eye & How Vision Works - Vision Center. https://www.visioncenter.org/eye-anatomy/.

[3] The structure of the eye (video) | Khan Academy. https://www.khanacademy.org/science/health-and-medicine/nervous-system-and-sensory-infor/sight-vision/v/vision-structure-of-the-eye.

[4] See Well for a Lifetime PARTS OF THE EYE - National Eye Institute. https://www.nei.nih.gov/sites/default/files/2019-05/EyeHandout_508.pdf.

[5] Emerging Strategies in Corneal Regeneration - American Academy of …. https://www.aao.org/eyenet/article/emerging-strategies-in-corneal-regeneration.

[6] Regenerating Eye Tissues to Preserve and Restore Vision - Cell Press. https://www.cell.com/cell-stem-cell/pdf/S1934-5909%2818%2930231-5.pdf.

[7] Regenerating optic pathways from the eye to the brain - Science. https://www.science.org/doi/epdf/10.1126/science.aal5060.

[8] 8 'Do Not Ignore' Warning Signs of Serious Eye Problems. https://www.optometrists.org/general-practice-optometry/guide-to-eye-health/8-do-not-ignore-warning-signs-of-serious-eye-problems/.

[9] Ocular Regenerative Medicine Institute | Harvard Medical School …. https://eye.hms.harvard.edu/ormi.

[10] The Eye and Immune Privilege - American Academy of Ophthalmology. https://www.aao.org/eye-health/tips-prevention/eye-immune-privilege.

[11] The protective mechanism in the Eye - OptomInSight - Optometryblogs. https://optominsight.com/eye-protective-mechanism/.

[12] Immune responses to injury and their links to eye disease. https://www.translationalres.com/article/S1931-5244%2821%2900123-7/pdf.

[13] Pathophysiology of Ocular Trauma | Clinical Gate. https://clinicalgate.com/pathophysiology-of-ocular-trauma/

16

John's Protocol

When I was first told that I had CRVO in September of 2016, I had great hope that I would be able to restore some of my vision or at least be able to stabilize the bleeding, but seven months later, that didn't happen. From the moment I was diagnosed until April 2017, there had not been any improvement at all. In fact, the condition of my eye appeared to be worsening. My ophthalmologist even informed me that by the way things were going, there was a high likelihood of CRVO developing in my left eye as well. I felt utterly hopeless and frightened. The black spot was getting bigger, and every doctor's visit showed a more significant leak. Furthermore, my situation was exacerbated by the onset of Posterior Vitreous Detachment (PVD) in the CRVO-affected eye, leading to extreme visual distortion.

One thing I had going for me was that I had just switched doctors and was now getting treated at one of the best eye institutions in the country. I was reassured that I was getting top-notch care. Yet, it was disheartening to discover that my new physician, much like the previous one, was just as short on answers about my condition. Every visit, they'd rush me in and rush me out after the injection. The only avenue for answers that I had was the information that resided on my fundus photos.

Fortunately, I seized every opportunity to capture snapshots of my eye scans, using my cellphone to take pictures of the computer screens. These images enabled me to monitor any changes in my eye's condition by comparing them with others from my past appointments. It wasn't much, but it was better than nothing, and I was grateful to have them. After each visit, I'd stare at these images, determined that I would see progress one day.

Then, one night in April of 2017, I noticed a physical change in my eye after eating a homemade Italian dinner. My eye had stopped twitching. An eye twitch is usually not considered a CRVO condition or side effect, but I had had it since the moment I was diagnosed with the eye stroke. I had even asked my ophthalmologist about it, and he suggested that it was probably due to the blood struggling to get through and that there was nothing I could do about it.

So, after dinner, I pondered what could have stopped the twitching. The meal was unassuming: pasta with tomato sauce and toast adorned with bruschetta made out of tomatoes, garlic, cilantro, salt, and pepper. I wondered if it could be the garlic. After all, I had finely chopped eight raw cloves and generously sprinkled them onto the bruschetta before crowning the toast with this flavorful mixture.

Curious, I hopped on my computer and did a search on the health benefits of raw garlic. What I found amazed me. While the rest of the world knew of its health benefits, I was clueless. I just loved its flavor—the more, the better, I figured. Who knew that its compounds would become my saving grace?

The Healing Power of Garlic

Raw garlic is renowned for its healing properties, which include a range of benefits from antioxidant, antifungal, antiviral, and antibacterial activities to potential cancer-fighting and immune-boosting effects[2]. Another key benefit is that it expands the blood vessels and also thins the blood[1].

So, when considering the doctor's explanation that the eye twitching was due to blood flow difficulties, it seems logical to deduce that when I consumed that large amount of garlic, it might have facilitated the blood's passage, leading to the cessation of my twitch. Studies have suggested that garlic's sulfur compounds, including allicin, can increase tissue blood flow and lower blood pressure by relaxing your blood vessels[3]. This vasodilation effect is beneficial for improving circulation and may contribute to the health benefits associated with garlic, including its impact on heart disease and arterial health[3][4].

Almost immediately after learning this, I wrote to my online CRVO group and told them what had happened. Then, I asked if anyone had had a similar experience with the healing powers of food that they noticed improved their vision or condition. Everyone said no, but then, this one lady sent me a private message saying she had heard about a painter who wrote a book on how he healed both his eyes from macular degeneration. She suggested that even though I didn't suffer from the same disease, the book might help, and then she sent me an Amazon link, and I bought it.

"Blind Faith: Reverse Macular Degeneration Through Diet & Nutrition" is penned by a Canadian artist named John Crittenden, who was diagnosed with macular degeneration in his right eye in 2011. In a matter of months, his vision deteriorated to the point of legal blindness, and he was told that his sight would not return. Then, the horrible condition began to affect his other eye. After two years of monthly injections of Avastin with no appreciable improvement, John embarked on a quest to unravel the reasons behind his deteriorating eyesight. In the process, he reversed his macular degeneration, which is not supposed to be possible, and then wrote a book on his protocol so that others could benefit from what he learned.

After reading the book, I didn't know what to think. Even if it were true, would his protocol help someone with CRVO? Plus, I had another problem—health insurance. While my insurance wasn't bad, it wasn't great and had high out-of-pocket costs. John had the luxury of using the Canadian healthcare system, where he and his doctors could order various types of blood work to monitor his progress, working together in tandem. In America, healthcare insurance companies limit what patients can test for, costs can triple outside the network, and in no way did my doctors appear interested in fixing my condition. As long as the injections stabilized the bleeding, they were happy. So, for about a month, I debated whether or not to give it a try. Then, during my May 15th ophthalmologist appointment, I decided to give it a shot after seeing my dismal fundus photos. My condition was getting worse.

To say I doubted the chances of John's protocol working for me was an understatement. After all, I didn't have macular degeneration, and without the means to measure nutrient deficiencies or track any improvement, I would be on my own. Yet, the protocol would only take eleven weeks, so what did I have to lose? Nothing.

So, the first step was deciphering John's book. To be honest, it's not an easy read. I often found myself lost in its technical passages and was stumped trying to find the exact supplements, vitamins, or components he used. However, I was able to wade through the complexities and reduce it to its essential elements.

Step One: Put the body in a state of healing

- Achieve an 8.0 pH Balance
- Enhance Gut Health
- Oxygenate the Cells
- Strengthen Cell Membranes

Step Two: Feed the body

- Vitamins, Supplements, and a Healthy Diet
- Maintain Cellular Voltage with Exercise and Sleep

Once I streamlined the process to align with John's protocol and ensured it was comprehensive, I ordered the necessary items from Amazon. As soon as they arrived, I wasted no time starting the regimen. After four weeks, my eyesight improved to 20/100, then at eight weeks, 20/50, and finally, at twelve weeks, my vision was restored to 20/30.

The prominent black spot persisted, but it started to lose its opacity, allowing me to see through it. So, for the first time in eleven months, I could actually see again.

Endnotes

[1] Raw Garlic: Healing Properties and Medicinal Uses. https://drfarrahmd.com/2021/04/raw-garlic-healing-properties-and/.

[2] Raw Garlic: Healing Properties and Medicinal Uses - HealWithFood.org. https://bing.com/search?q=healing+power+of+raw+garlic.

[3] The 13 Best Foods to Increase Blood Flow and Circulation - Healthline. https://www.healthline.com/nutrition/foods-that-increase-blood-flow.

[4] Natural vasodilators: How to dilate blood vessels naturally and .... https://www.belmarrahealth.com/natural-vasodilators-dilate-blood-vessels-naturally-increase-blood-flow/.

[5] Crittenden, John. BLIND FAITH: The Incredible Story of a Professional Artist Who Overcame Blindness Through Diet & Nutrition

Visit John's Website

Before I dive into my journey of healing my eyesight and improving my CRVO condition, I'd like to note that I won't be delving deeply into the full intricacies of John Crittenden's method. However, I do outline the key parts of the protocol with brief explanations for each component.

If you wish to learn more about the specific steps he took to heal his body or the complexities of his discoveries, theories, and findings, I highly recommend visiting his website or purchasing his book, Blind Faith: Reverse Macular Degeneration Through Diet & Nutrition.

Blind Faith is available on his website, Amazon, and most online bookstores.

www.johncrittenden.com

3 STEPS OF HEALING

17

The Game Plan

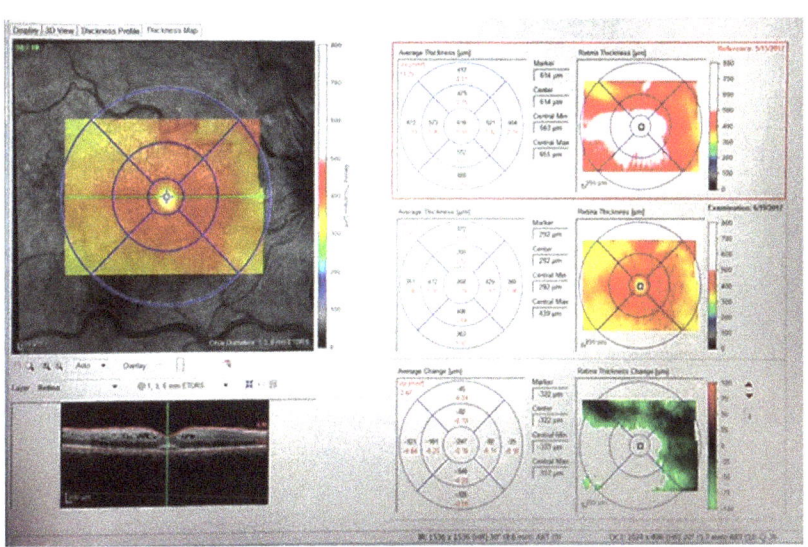

To my relief, John's protocol worked. My vision improved drastically. Don't get me wrong, it was still bad, but so much better.

I couldn't believe it. I was so excited. Yet, as soon as I stopped doing the protocol, the leaking in my eye returned, swelling my macula. At that moment, I realized that CRVO stems from multiple factors, and in order to heal, each one needs to be dealt with on its own. There were three things I had never considered before, and they were:

- #1: The injections only stop the bleeding.
- #2: The protocol only repairs the eye.
- #3: Ugh, I wasn't doing anything for the blockage!

How could that be?

After all, I did have an eye stroke, which is similar to a brain stroke. So, why weren't my doctors doing some kind of tests to monitor the blockage or giving me some sort of drug to deal with it? When I asked my ophthalmologist about it, he advised me to consult my general practitioner.

However, when I approached my GP, he simply shrugged and mentioned that an eye stroke doesn't pose an immediate life-threatening risk, and because I didn't have heart disease, there were no specific tests or treatments available.

Faced with the reality of my situation, it became evident that I would need to take matters into my own hands if I wanted to fully heal from this ugly disease, and I devised a game plan.

First, I broke the healing process down into three components:

STEP 1: Stop the Leak
STEP 2: Repair the Eye
STEP 3: Unblock the Blockage

It's essential to recognize that you'll likely be tackling all three steps simultaneously. I've listed them in order of importance. The top priority is halting the growth of abnormal blood vessels to minimize eye damage.

Next up is repairing the eye's cells and rods, and lastly, unblocking the blockage. This final step is the most gradual, as it demands lifestyle changes and, in some cases, medication.

After mapping out my game plan, I meticulously reviewed all my CRVO fundus images, pored over my notes, and sifted through my memories to pinpoint the exact dates and times of my most severe CRVO leaks. I retraced my steps to recall what might have triggered each incident.

I then scoured the web, read countless books, and watched numerous videos to grasp the eye's healing process and discover ways to unblock arteries. I explored the benefits of specific foods, sleep patterns, and physical exercises for both the eyes and body, pursuing every promising lead that could enhance the CRVO healing process.

Most importantly, I embraced those spontaneous flashes of insight or epiphanies that visited me in the wee hours of the night, sparking breakthroughs when least expected.

The process, in truth, isn't overly complex, but it does call for daily dedication, lifestyle adjustments, and mindfulness. In the next three chapters, I'll break down each component in detail, sharing various healing methods as well as my personal strategies, insights, and the ways I tackled them.

18

Step 1: Stop the Leak

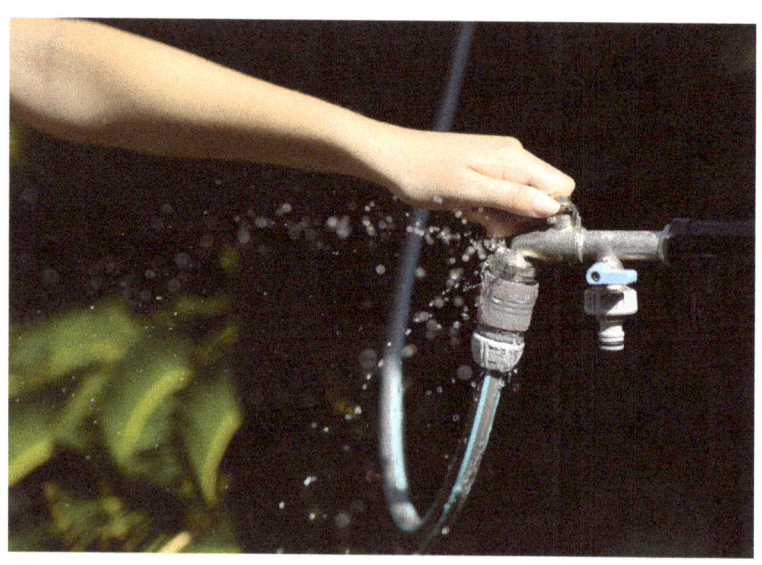

First things first, how do you determine if your eye is leaking blood between injections? In my situation, often, after a workout, my vision would blur with a pinkish tint, prompting me to wonder if my eye was leaking, though I couldn't exactly tell at the moment.

However, my fears were almost always confirmed the following morning when I woke to extremely blotchy and blurry vision. Interestingly, I was never 100% positive because, as the day wore on, my vision would get clearer, which left me confused.

My ophthalmologist suggested that this could be happening because I slept on my back, causing the blood leaking from abnormal blood vessels to shift and cover my optic nerve, which provides vision. However, due to gravity, the blood would collect at the bottom of the eye as I sat or stood during the day until the body absorbed it.

In my early days, it would freak me out because I thought that while I slept, my eye was getting worse. Thankfully, that wasn't the case. Sometimes, the leaks are very mild at first, and then your vision gets progressively blurrier as the days go by.

The abnormal blood vessels in a CRVO eye are like a finicky garden hose—when the pressure is just right, everything stays dry. But crank up the hydraulic force, and suddenly, you've got a watery mess. Similarly, keeping your blood pressure low helps prevent those pesky abnormal blood vessels from growing and leaking into the eye.

The most terrifying blood-leaking episode I had ever experienced occurred in December 2016. My eye doctor had rescheduled my usual four-week injection to six weeks due to her holiday plans. At the time, I was thrilled, thinking my eye must be doing better for her to delay it because I had been leaking every four weeks to the day.

Furthermore, I was also going away for the holidays and was worried about traveling with CRVO, so I asked her if it was okay to fly. She just smiled at me and then, with her high-pitched laugh, told me I didn't have a thing to worry about.

STEP 1: STOP THE LEAK

Well, once again, she was wrong. By the time my flight landed in New York, my black spot had turned blotchy red, and my eye was throbbing.

Honestly, I couldn't tell you if it was due to my blood pressure rising as I carried my luggage to and from the bag drop-off or if it was due to the plane's cabin pressure at the high altitudes, but what I can say is that my Fitbit recorded my highest BPM mid-flight.

To say my holidays were ruined goes without saying. I was so frightened to move or do anything that would exacerbate my condition. The next ten days felt like an eternity as I waited for my doctor to return from her vacation so that I could get an emergency appointment with her to get the injection.

Needless to say, my doctor should have known better and been more vigilant in either administering the Avastin injection within my 4-5 week timeframe or she should have referred me to a colleague for treatment. Her complete lack of regard for my well-being left me with no other choice but to find a more experienced ophthalmologist.

On a positive note, the frightening experience underscored the significance of timely CRVO treatments.

Do NOT miss an injection!

Skipping recommended intravitreal injections will only make your eye condition worse. I have to admit that when I was first diagnosed with CRVO, I looked for every reason possible to avoid getting an injection. I hated them with a passion. If my doctor told me I didn't need one, I would feel elated, filled with hope that my eye was healing, only to discover, a week or two later, that it was leaking more than ever.

STEP 1: STOP THE LEAK

As the years went by and my CRVO eye healed, I realized that the injections were crucial for me to maintain a normal lifestyle. It was also at that point that I realized that I needed to analyze my daily routine to figure out why my eye was leaking so badly in between injections.

Then, one day at the gym, I noticed my vision becoming blurry while I was lifting weights. I knew instantly that this was the culprit, which confused me because both of my doctors told me I could exercise normally without worrying about my eye leaking.

So, were my doctors correct in saying I could work out the same as if I didn't have CRVO? Well, yes and no because exercise does play a vital role in maintaining and improving the eye's health, and many exercises are safe for CRVO patients. Yet, there are a handful that should be avoided or monitored closely.

In my situation, I discovered that when I didn't pay attention to certain types of strenuous exercise, such as weightlifting, yoga, and certain aerobic activities, my CRVO eye would blur. Which almost always led to a massive blowout of my vision the following morning from the leakage and would put my life on hold until I could get an injection.

Most CRVO patients are unaware that every time their eye leaks, it sets their healing process back weeks or months, so it is best to prevent or avoid the leakage from happening in the first place.

Upon discovering that my exercise routine was triggering many of my eye leaks, I decided to take a proactive approach. I invested in a better exercise watch capable of monitoring my BPM and any irregular rhythms, allowing me to keep a close eye on my heart rate and better manage my workouts to prevent further issues.

STEP 1: STOP THE LEAK

At the time, I was getting Eylea injections, which typically last 6 to 8 weeks in the eye. Knowing this, I determined that I needed to lighten my workouts during the first week of my injections, resume normal workouts from weeks two to five, and then dial the workout down again during weeks six through eight as the medicine's effects began to wane.

The blurring of my vision was my gauge

The process took months of trial and error, accompanied by numerous eye leaks, to uncover my limits. Ultimately, I discovered that if my BPM exceeded 110, my vision would blur. My weightlifting had to be restricted to 20-30 lbs with slow, controlled reps. At any sign of tension in my eye, I would dial back and opt for lighter reps or reduce the speed. On the treadmill or exercise bike, I had to maintain a gentle, steady pace to prevent further issues.

Exercise is very important to healing the body and the eyes and should not be avoided. I realize that some of you might be thinking that if exercising is causing your eye to leak, then stop doing it. However, staying active can play a pivotal role in managing various eye conditions. By engaging in regular physical activity, you boost your overall vascular health, which is key to maintaining your eye health. Plus, exercise also gives your body the energy needed to repair itself.

Here are some ways exercise can help:

1. Improves Blood Circulation: Exercise promotes better blood flow, which can help deliver essential nutrients and oxygen to the eyes.

2. Reduces Intraocular Pressure: Activities like walking or moderate aerobic exercise can help lower intraocular pressure, which is beneficial for conditions like glaucoma.

3. Prevents Eye Diseases: Studies suggest that regular exercise may reduce the risk of developing serious eye diseases such as age-related macular degeneration (AMD) and diabetic retinopathy.

4. Manages Systemic Conditions: Exercise helps control conditions like diabetes and high blood pressure, which can have a significant impact on eye health.

But remember, it's important to consult with your physician before starting any new exercise regimen, especially if you have an eye condition like CRVO. Your doctor can help tailor an exercise plan that is safe and effective for your specific needs.

Safe Exercises for CRVO patients

1. Walking: A low-impact activity that can improve circulation without straining your eyes. Aim for a brisk pace to get your heart rate up.

2. Swimming: This is an excellent full-body workout that is gentle on the eyes and helps improve cardiovascular health.

3. Cycling: Stationary biking or gentle outdoor cycling can be effective in maintaining fitness without putting excessive pressure on the eyes.

4. Stretching and Flexibility Exercises: Incorporate gentle stretching and flexibility exercises to keep your muscles limber and promote blood flow.

5. Tai Chi: This ancient Chinese practice involves slow, controlled movements and

STEP 1: STOP THE LEAK

deep breathing, which can help improve balance, flexibility, and circulation.

6. Yoga (without inversions): Gentle yoga poses can help reduce stress, improve flexibility, and promote relaxation without straining the eyes.

7. Eye Exercises: Using an eye exercise app like *Vision Workout: Eye Training from Sports Vision Training*[5] for just a couple of minutes a day can significantly improve your eye health and vision. Look for an app that includes exercises where your eyes follow an object moving in various directions, such as up and down or side to side. Regular use can help in enhancing your eye's condition and overall vision clarity. During my PVD episode, I used several apps on my iPhone that worked great. The PVD caused my vision to become distorted, but daily and weekly exercises helped restore it. You can find these apps in your phone's app store.

Exercises To Monitor

Weight Lifting:

Navigating the world of weightlifting with CRVO requires extra care. While regular exercise boosts overall health, heavy lifting can ramp up intraocular pressure, straining your eyes and potentially worsening the condition. If you're determined to lift weights, do so mindfully, always keeping an eye on your vision. Hit the pause button at the slightest hint of blurring or tension in your affected eye. Also, continuous breathing during weightlifting relieves eye pressure. Personally, I dial down the weights until I reach a point where my eyes feel no strain. You can lift weights, but be careful.

Yoga:

While yoga can be very beneficial for CRVO patients, certain poses can be risky, particularly those that cause the head to drop below the heart, leading to a rush of blood. Over the years, I have experienced a few leaks after intense yoga classes. Generally, yoga is considered safe for managing CRVO, but it's important to be cautious. Some yoga poses, especially those involving inversions or significant straining moves, might increase intraocular pressure and potentially worsen your condition by raising your blood pressure.

Avoid Yoga Poses like:

- Headstands
- Shoulder stands
- Downward-facing dog

Focus on gentle, low-impact poses that promote relaxation and circulation without straining the eyes. Overall, yoga is considered safe for managing CRVO, and you shouldn't avoid it because it has so many health benefits, especially for older adults, but it's important to be cautious.

Here are some simple eye yoga exercises that you can do while relaxing or watching TV:

1. Palming (Trataka): Rub your palms together to create warmth, then gently place them over your closed eyes without pressing. Breathe deeply and relax, focusing on the warmth.

2. Eye Rolling: Sit comfortably and slowly roll your eyes in a clockwise direction, then switch to counterclockwise. This helps stimulate circulation around the eyes.

3. Focus Shifting (Nasikagra Drishti): Extend one arm forward and make a gentle fist with your thumb facing upward. Focus on your thumb and slowly bring it towards your nose, then extend your arm again.

4. Upward and Downward Gazing (Urdhva Drishti): Sit in a relaxed position and slowly look upward as far as you can, then look downward. Repeat this movement five times each way, focusing on deep breaths.

STEP 1: STOP THE LEAK

5. Blinking: In a comfortable position, blink your eyes quickly for 20 seconds, then close and relax them.

Running:

In my CRVO group, a young man from India reached out, sharing that he had been following my protocol but noticed his CRVO eye worsening. Curious, I asked if he was exercising, to which he replied that he was simply running. It turned out that he was training for a marathon. He had been assured by his doctor that it wouldn't harm his condition. I advised him to start monitoring his BPM while running to check if it was too high, and in the end, it turned out to be the culprit.

Running is great for overall health, but if you're dealing with CRVO (Central Retinal Vein Occlusion), a bit of caution goes a long way. High-impact activities like running can elevate intraocular pressure and place undue strain on the eyes. Marathon-level exertion? Probably not the best idea. The intense and sustained effort might worsen eye conditions by increasing intraocular pressure.

It is important to note that each of us is different and that we each have different thresholds. In order to stop the leaking, it is essential that you first figure out what is causing it and then figure out what your limits are.

Can certain foods cause eye leaks?

While there isn't strong evidence directly linking specific foods to eye leaks in CRVO patients, maintaining a healthy diet is crucial for overall eye health and managing conditions like CRVO. Some dietary factors that can help improve your condition include:

- Anti-inflammatory Foods: Incorporating fruits and vegetables rich in vitamins A, C, and potassium, along with polyphenols and carotenoids, can help reduce inflammation and support eye health.

- Balanced Diet: A diet rich in fiber, omega-3 fatty acids, and antioxidants can promote vascular health and reduce the risk of complications.

- Avoid Excessive Sodium and Sugar: High amounts of either can contribute to hypertension and bloating, which may exacerbate CRVO symptoms.

Can sleep cause CRVO eye leaks?

Sleep is needed to repair the eyes, but sleep itself doesn't directly cause CRVO eye leaks. However, certain factors related to sleep, such as changes in blood pressure and eye pressure during sleep, could potentially contribute to eye strain or exacerbate existing conditions. It's important to maintain a healthy sleep routine and consult with your healthcare provider if you notice any changes in your eye health.

Endnote:

[1] Exercise for Eyes and Vision. https://www.aao.org/eye-health/diseases/exercise-eyes-vision-4

[2] Intense Exercise Causing Central Retinal Vein Occlusion in a Young Patient: Case Report and Review of the Literature. https://pmc.ncbi.nlm.nih.gov/articles/PMC4025055/

[3] Prevention and Treatment of Retinal Vein Occlusion: The Role of Diet—A Review. https://pmc.ncbi.nlm.nih.gov/articles/PMC10383741/

[4] Central Retinal Vein Occlusion Recovery: Pathways to Improved Vision. https://armadale-eye.com.au/central-retinal-vein-occlusion-recovery/

[5] 11 Best Eye Exercise Apps (Android & iOS). https://freeappsforme.com/eye-exercise-apps/

Stop the Leak Summary

1. Get your eye injection when scheduled.

2. Monitor your blood pressure, and check your heart rate (BPM) during workouts.

3. Avoid high-impact activities that can elevate your intraocular pressure and strain your eyes.

4. Follow a low-impact exercise regimen and avoid overexertion that could cause your blood pressure to rise.

5. Stop immediately if you experience blurred vision while working out or exercising.

6. Avoid inflammatory foods, drink plenty of water, and reduce excessive sugar and sodium intake.

7. Get a good night's sleep.

19

Step 2: Repair the Eye

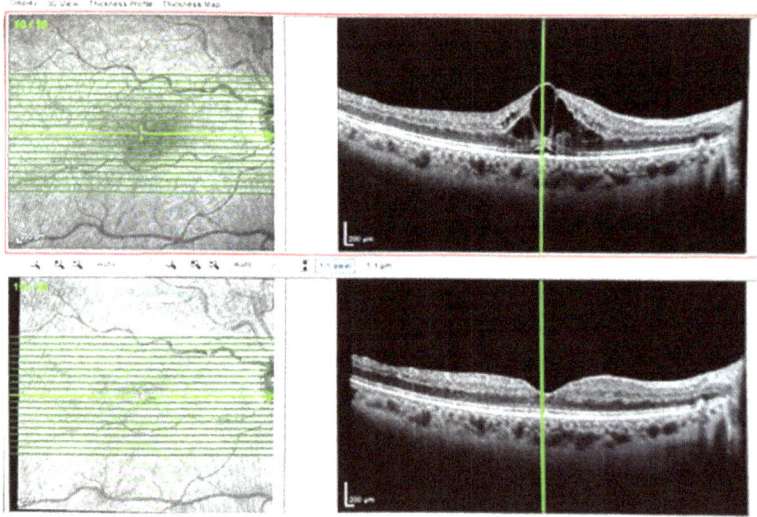

In *Blind Faith: Reverse Macular Degeneration Thru Diet & Nutrition*, the author, John Crittenden, suggests that the body grows new retinal elements (rods and cones) every two days and goes on further to suggest that each new cell that is built requires certain nutrients and other building materials to facilitate

STEP 2: REPAIR THE EYE

its creation. The body's healing and regenerative process is truly amazing. But, just like a well-oiled machine needs fuel and maintenance to work correctly, so do our bodies require a steady supply of nutrients, exercise, and sleep to facilitate the process.

With this knowledge and the realization that the human eye suffers from immune privilege (Chapter 15), John realized that the only way to heal his eyes from macular degeneration was to heal the overall body. In the end, he determined that there were eight critical stages that were needed to achieve this goal[1]:

1. Oxygenate the cells
2. Maintain correct cellular voltage
3. Build up body electrons
4. Get enough minerals and vitamins
5. Maintain sufficient stomach acid
6. Get adequate sleep
7. Eliminate chronic inflammation
8. Eliminate chronic calcification

Once again, since I didn't have access to the same type of healthcare and doctors that John did, which would allow me to monitor which nutrients I was missing, I simplified the process to just the elements that he used in his protocol.

The basic concept of John Crittenden's Protocol is to put the body in a state of healing by making it more alkaline, based on the idea that an acidic environment can hinder nutrient absorption. Then, the body is provided with the needed nutrients, exercise, and sufficient sleep for a duration of eleven weeks.

Here is the regimen structure and breakdown of the elements in John's protocol:

- **Sodium Bicarbonate (Baking Soda):** Take 1/2 teaspoon daily to temporarily maintain a pH of 8.0 and ensure proper cellular voltage, aiding the body in producing healthy, functioning cells. Follow a cycle of two weeks on, one week off, repeated for eleven weeks. Monitoring using pH strips daily is essential[1].

STEP 2: REPAIR THE EYE

- **Nurture Stomach Acid Levels:** Enhance your digestion with Betaine and/or Probiotics as needed to ensure optimal digestion and nutrient absorption[1].

- **Evening Primrose Oil (Omega 6):** Take 4 grams daily throughout the duration of the protocol to support cellular oxygenation[1].

- **Flax Seed Oil (Omega 3):** Take 1 gram daily to fortify your cell membranes with the nourishment they need to stay healthy and strong[1].

- **Vitamins & Minerals:** These nutrients are vital to our bodies, and, much like oxygen, we cannot do without them. They weave their way into our lives through both organic and inorganic forms and are found in the foods we eat or supplements we take[1]. For John's protocol, he and his doctors determined what his body needed. In my case, I simply took a multivitamin that contained a potent mix of 23 vitamins and minerals, including high-potency B vitamins such as B12 and folate, as well as vitamins A, C, D3, E, biotin, and zinc.

- **Build Up Body Electrons:** Essential for energy. Harness electrons through exercise and grounding—powerful methods of charging your body's energy stores. Ensure sufficient stomach acid to aid in this process[1].

- **Get adequate sleep:** Scientific research suggests that the body undergoes significant regeneration and cell repair during the night when minimal energy is expended on other activities. As a result, it is recommended that the protocol be done every evening.

- **Eliminate Chronic Inflammation & Calcification:** Many medical conditions and diseases share a common thread: inflammation and calcification. By tackling these chronic conditions head-on, CRVO patients can significantly improve their healing potential and pave the way for better outcomes.

STEP 2: REPAIR THE EYE

For most CRVO sufferers, there are likely untapped opportunities to enhance their well-being. Whether it's refining their diet, incorporating essential nutrients, embracing regular exercise, or exploring medication, small changes can lead to significant improvements.

Overview of the Components

Why Sodium Bicarbonate (Baking Soda)?

John suggests that Sodium Bicarbonate (Baking Soda) might just be one of the world's most extraordinary substances, being incredibly versatile and safe. It is a natural compound found throughout nature and is highly beneficial in treating various diseases, including cancer and kidney diseases. Unlike harmful chemical compounds, baking soda does not negatively affect us or the environment. Its neutralizing properties make it extremely helpful as a medicine, especially in our current age of increased toxicity[1].

Sodium bicarbonate (baking soda) helps to make your body more alkaline by neutralizing excess stomach acid. When ingested, it reacts with hydrochloric acid in the stomach to form sodium chloride (table salt), water, and carbon dioxide. This reaction increases the pH level in your stomach, making it less acidic.

However, it's important to note that this effect is temporary and primarily occurs in the stomach. The body's overall pH balance is tightly regulated by various systems, and ingesting baking soda is not a reliable way to significantly alter your body's pH levels.

Why Nurture Stomach Acid Levels?

Probiotics can be used to nurture stomach acid levels and support overall digestive health. John suggests that stomach acid is like the unsung hero in our body's healing and cell regeneration journey. It plays a crucial role in the body's ability to heal and regenerate new cells[1]. Here's how:

STEP 2: REPAIR THE EYE

1. Digestion and Absorption: Stomach acid helps break down food into smaller, absorbable components, including proteins into amino acids. These amino acids are essential for cell repair and growth[17].

2. Defense Mechanism: Stomach acid acts as a barrier, killing harmful bacteria and pathogens that enter the digestive system and preventing infections that could hinder healing[17].

3. Cell Proliferation: Proper levels of stomach acid are necessary for the proliferation of epithelial cells in the stomach lining, which is vital for healing ulcers and other injuries[17].

4. Growth Factors: Stomach acid helps activate certain growth factors and enzymes that promote tissue repair and regeneration[17].

Certain probiotic strains, such as Lactobacillus and Bifidobacterium, are naturally resistant to stomach acid and can survive the journey to the intestines, where they confer health benefits. Taking probiotics on an empty stomach or with meals that contain fats can also improve their survival rates[17]. However, imbalances in stomach acid levels can lead to issues. Low stomach acid can result in poor digestion and nutrient absorption, affecting the body's ability to heal. On the other hand, high stomach acid can cause damage to the stomach lining, leading to ulcers and other issues that impede healing.

Why Evening Primrose Oil (Omega 6)?

John suggests that all diseases are linked to a lack of oxygen at the cellular level. Scientific research emphasizes the crucial role of intracellular oxygen in maintaining good health. To ensure our cells are optimally oxygenated, we must avoid oxygen-resistive oils like canola oil and other highly processed vegetable oils and instead embrace oxygen-enabling oils known as Parent Essential Oils[1][3].

STEP 2: REPAIR THE EYE

Here are some Parent Essential Oils:

- Avocado Oil
- Evening primrose Oil
- Flaxseed Oil
- Pumpkin Seed Oil
- Safflower Oil
- Sunflower Seed Oil
- Walnut Oil

Professor Brian S. Peskin has written books on Parent Essential Oils (PEOs) and passionately emphasizes that our bodies are composed of 100 trillion cells, each with a membrane—over 30% of which are made up of polyunsaturated fatty acids. He advocates for the consumption of Parent Essential Oils, which are adept at attracting oxygen and integrating into our cell membranes, thereby facilitating high levels of oxygen transfer from the blood into our cells. He warns against the consumption of modern vegetable oils, especially after they've been heated, as they severely hinder oxygen absorption, ultimately leading to cellular death[1][3].

The Crittenden Protocol addresses 'oxygen-starved cells' by providing continuous oxygen directly to the cells. It replaces harmful vegetable oils in the cells with oxygen-carrying Parent Essential Oils, such as Evening Primrose Oil and Safflower Oil. This process allows cells to breathe, absorb nutrients, and eliminate waste, fostering a healthy environment for normal oxygen transfer from the blood to the cells[1].

Why Flaxseed Oil (Omega 3)?

John utilizes flaxseed oil in his protocol because it is a rich source of omega-3 fatty acids, specifically alpha-linolenic acid (ALA), which is essential for maintaining cell membrane integrity and fluidity[1]. Omega-3 fatty acids help reduce inflammation and support overall cell function, contributing to healthier cells, which is crucial for maintaining heart health and promoting overall well-being. He also suggests not using fish oil as a supplement for omega-3 due to potential health risks[1].

It's important to note that there is a proper omega-6 to omega-3 ratio that needs to be maintained. Our tissues and organs with Parent Essential Oils need significantly more unadulterated omega-6 than omega-3 to function properly. The ideal ratio of "good" omega-6 to omega-3 is between 7:1 and 8.5:1. This higher ratio of omega-6 helps the "good" omega-6 combat and overpower the "bad" omega-6, providing the necessary protection for our bodies. Together, both omega-3 and omega-6 provide the body with a balance of cellular oxygen and support for cell membranes.

Why Vitamins & Minerals?

In John's book, the author discusses the various ways we obtain minerals, vitamins, amino acids, and antioxidants and also points out deficiencies that may arise from our food intake or genetic makeup. There are two types of vitamins: water-soluble and fat-soluble. The main difference between the two is how they are absorbed, stored, and excreted by the body. Here is an overview of vitamins and minerals[1].

Vitamins

1) Water-soluble vitamins

Water-soluble vitamins are a group of vitamins that dissolve in water and are not stored in large amounts in the body. This means they need to be consumed regularly in the diet to maintain adequate levels. These vitamins are easily excreted through urine, which reduces the risk of toxicity but also means they can be quickly depleted[18].

The primary water-soluble vitamins are:

- Vitamin C (Ascorbic Acid): Important for the growth and repair of tissues, immune function, and antioxidant protection.

Found in citrus fruits (oranges, lemons), strawberries, bell peppers, broccoli, Brussels sprouts, and spinach[18].

B-Complex Vitamins [18]:

- B1 (Thiamine): Essential for energy metabolism and nerve function. Found in whole grains, meat (especially pork), fish, seeds, nuts, and legumes.

- B2 (Riboflavin): Plays a key role in energy production and skin health. Found in eggs, lean meats, milk, green vegetables, and fortified cereals.

- B3 (Niacin): Important for digestive health, skin health, and converting food into energy. Found in poultry, fish, lean meats, peanuts, and legumes.

- B5 (Pantothenic Acid): Vital for the synthesis of coenzyme A and energy metabolism. Found in chicken, beef, potatoes, oats, tomatoes, and whole grains.

- B6 (Pyridoxine): Involved in amino acid metabolism, red blood cell production, and neurotransmitter synthesis. Found in fish, beef liver, potatoes, and non-citrus fruits like bananas and avocados.

- B7 (Biotin): Necessary for carbohydrate, fat, and protein metabolism, as well as maintaining healthy hair and nails. Found in eggs, almonds, spinach, sweet potatoes, and dairy products.

- B9 (Folate or Folic Acid): Crucial for DNA synthesis, cell division, and fetal development during pregnancy. Found in dark leafy greens, beans, peanuts, sunflower seeds, and liver.

- B12 (Cobalamin): Important for red blood cell formation, neurological function, and DNA synthesis. Found in fish, meat, poultry, eggs, milk, and other dairy products.

Since these vitamins are not stored in the body, it's important to include them in your daily diet through a variety of foods such as fruits, vegetables, whole grains, and lean proteins or by taking supplements.

2) Fat-soluble vitamins

Fat-soluble vitamins are a group of vitamins that dissolve in fat and are stored in the body's fatty tissue and liver. Because they can be stored, they don't need to be consumed as frequently as water-soluble vitamins. However, this also means they can accumulate to potentially toxic levels if taken in excessive amounts[18].

The primary fat-soluble vitamins are:

- Vitamin A: Important for vision, immune function, and skin health. Found in liver, fish oils, milk, eggs, and colorful fruits and vegetables (as beta-carotene, a precursor to vitamin A)[18].

- Vitamin D: Essential for calcium absorption and bone health. It also plays a role in immune function. Found in fatty fish, liver, egg yolks, and fortified foods. It is also produced by the skin in response to sunlight[18].

- Vitamin E: Acts as an antioxidant, protecting cells from damage caused by free radicals. Found in nuts, seeds, vegetable oils, and green leafy vegetables[18].

- Vitamin K: Crucial for blood clotting and bone health. Found in green leafy vegetables, such as kale and spinach, as well as in some vegetable oils and fermented foods[18].

In the book, John suggests that when the body doesn't have the nutrients it needs, it will grab the next best thing it has and use that to try to repair the damaged cells[1]. He also points out that if we have multiple health issues, we may need to take more of certain vitamins or minerals to heal or repair them.

Upon reading that and knowing that I wouldn't have a doctor telling me which nutrients I was deficient in, I chose Nature's Way Alive! Max3 Potency Adult Complete Multivitamin for my version of the protocol. This multivitamin is balanced and, in some cases, contains more than the daily requirement of certain nutrients. It is important to note that some vitamins can be toxic and even dangerous if not taken in the proper ratio. Here is a list of the toxic danger zones to watch out for:

Toxic vitamins when taken at high doses:

- Vitamin A: Excessive intake can lead to liver damage, headaches, dizziness, nausea, and even coma[6].

- Vitamin D: Overconsumption can cause hypercalcemia (high levels of calcium in the blood), leading to kidney stones, bone pain, and calcification of organs[6].

- Vitamin E: High doses can interfere with blood clotting and increase the risk of hemorrhage[6].

- Vitamin K: While toxicity is rare, extremely high doses can cause liver damage and affect blood clotting[6].

- Vitamin B6: Excessive amounts can lead to nerve damage, causing numbness and tingling in the limbs[6].

- Vitamin C: Overconsumption can cause nausea, diarrhea, and stomach cramps. Extremely high doses may also increase the risk of kidney stones[6].

*Important Warning about B-Complex Vitamins

For patients with CRVO, it's important to be cautious with certain vitamins, particularly Vitamin B12. Studies have shown that Vitamin B12 deficiency is common in CRVO patients and can negatively impact their clinical outcomes[7]. However, excessive intake of Vitamin B12 should also be avoided as it can lead to mild side effects like diarrhea and itching.

Additionally, B vitamins can be dangerous if taken in excessive amounts and may contribute to heart disease[8]. Specifically, excess niacin (Vitamin B3) has been linked to an increased risk of cardiovascular disease. High levels of niacin can lead to vascular inflammation, which can cause blood vessel damage and atherosclerosis (plaque buildup in arteries), increasing the risk of heart attack and stroke[8]. Once again, it is important to take B vitamins in their proper ratio.

Minerals

The body requires a variety of essential minerals to function properly, and they play a crucial role in supporting overall eye health and managing conditions like CRVO (Central Retinal Vein Occlusion). Here are some key minerals that can be beneficial[18].

- Calcium: Important for eye health, bone and teeth, muscle function, and nerve signaling. Found in dairy products (milk, cheese, yogurt), leafy green vegetables (kale, broccoli), fortified foods (orange juice, cereals), and fish with edible bones (sardines, salmon)[18].

- Phosphorus: Works with calcium to build strong bones and teeth and is involved in energy production. Found in meat, fish, poultry, eggs, dairy products, nuts, seeds, and whole grains[18].

- Potassium: Helps regulate fluid balance, muscle contractions, and nerve signals. Found in bananas, oranges, potatoes, sweet potatoes, spinach, tomatoes, beans, and peas[18].

- Sodium: Essential for maintaining fluid balance, nerve function, and muscle contractions. Found in table salt, processed foods, canned soups, and snacks (like chips and pretzels)[18].

- Magnesium: Helps improve blood flow and reduce inflammation. Involved in over 300 biochemical reactions in the body, including energy production and muscle function. Found in nuts (almonds, cashews), seeds (pumpkin, flax), whole grains, leafy green vegetables, and dark chocolate[18].

- Iron: Necessary for the production of hemoglobin, which carries oxygen in the blood. Found in red meat, poultry, fish, lentils, beans, tofu, spinach, and fortified cereals[18].

- Zinc: Supports the immune system and may help reduce the risk of macular degeneration. Found in meat, shellfish, dairy products, legumes (beans, chickpeas, lentils), seeds, nuts, and whole grains[18].

- Copper: Helps with iron absorption and is important for heart and nervous system health. Found in shellfish, nuts, seeds, whole-grain products, beans, and organ meats (liver)[18].

- Iodine: Essential for thyroid hormone production, which regulates metabolism. Found in seafood, dairy products, iodized salt, eggs, and some types of bread[18].

- Selenium: Acts as an antioxidant and supports immune function. Found in Brazil nuts, seafood, meat, eggs, and whole grains[18].

- Manganese: Involved in bone formation, blood clotting, and reducing inflammation. Found in whole grains, nuts, leafy green vegetables, tea, and legumes[18].

Just like vitamins, these minerals are obtained through a balanced diet that includes a variety of foods such as fruits, vegetables, whole grains, and lean proteins or by taking supplements[18].

Toxic minerals when taken at high doses

- Iron: Too much iron can cause organ damage, particularly to the liver and heart, and can be fatal in severe cases[6].

- Zinc: Excessive zinc can lead to nausea, vomiting, loss of appetite, and impaired immune function[6].

- Selenium: High doses can cause hair loss, gastrointestinal upset, fatigue, and nerve damage[6].

It's important to stick to the recommended daily allowances (RDAs) and consult with a healthcare provider before taking high doses of any supplements.

Why Build Up Body Electrons?

Grounding, also known as earthing, is a practice that involves reconnecting with the earth to harness its natural electric charge. The idea is that direct physical contact with the earth—such as walking barefoot on grass, sand, or soil—helps to balance the body's electrical energy and improve overall health[1][4].

In Blind Faith, John emphasizes the crucial role of exercise in generating energy and electrons, which are vital for the body's healing process. He highlights that both exercise and grounding are key methods for acquiring these essential electrons.

While it's a complex topic with entire books written about it, it's essential to note that we get electrons from the earth. They are vital for life, health, healing, and cell growth. Voltage represents the stored potential energy required for cells to function, while amperage refers to the movement of electrons performing work. Low voltage in the body leads to cellular issues, which worsen as the voltage (pH) decreases[1].

The key benefits of grounding include:

- Reducing Inflammation: By neutralizing free radicals, grounding can help decrease inflammation in the body[4].

- Improving Sleep: Many people report better sleep quality and reduced insomnia after regular grounding[4].

- Enhancing Mood: Grounding can promote a sense of calm and reduce feelings of stress and anxiety[4].

- Boosting Energy Levels: Reconnecting with the earth may increase energy and vitality[4].

The science behind grounding suggests that the earth's surface has a negative charge, which can help balance the positive charge in our bodies caused by modern living and exposure to electronic devices [4].

Why Eliminate Chronic Calcification?

Taking too many calcium supplements can lead to hypercalcemia (high blood calcium levels), which can cause symptoms like bone pain, fatigue, frequent urination, and even kidney stones[10]. Excessive calcium can also increase the risk of heart disease and cognitive decline[9].

Effects on the Brain and Eyes:

Chronic calcification, particularly in the pineal gland, has a significant impact on melatonin production. High levels of calcium can negatively impact brain health, potentially leading to cognitive decline and memory problems. On the other hand, melatonin supports brain health by regulating sleep and reducing oxidative stress[13]. Adequate melatonin levels are also linked to better eye health and may help prevent age-related vision loss.

STEP 2: REPAIR THE EYE

Why Eliminate Chronic Inflammation?

Eliminating chronic inflammation is crucial for CRVO patients because inflammation can exacerbate the condition and lead to further complications. Chronic inflammation can contribute to macular edema (swelling of the macula), which is a common cause of vision loss in CRVO patients. By reducing inflammation, patients can potentially improve their overall eye health and slow the progression of the disease[16]. To reduce inflammation in CRVO patients, here are some strategies:

- Anti-inflammatory Medications: Corticosteroids and non-steroidal anti-inflammatory drugs (NSAIDs) can help reduce inflammation and swelling in the eye[16].

- Healthy Diet: Consuming a diet rich in fruits, vegetables, and omega-3 fatty acids can support overall eye health and reduce inflammation[16].

- Regular Exercise: Gentle, low-impact exercises like walking and swimming can improve circulation and reduce inflammation[16].

- Avoid Smoking: Smoking can damage blood vessels and increase inflammation, so quitting smoking is crucial for eye health[16].

- Manage Stress: Stress can exacerbate inflammation, so practices like yoga, meditation, and mindfulness can be beneficial.

Repair the Eye Summary

As you can see, many factors contribute to and combat a disease like Central Retinal Vein Occlusion, but don't worry. You do not have to get bogged down in the complexity. I've included an easy-to-follow list on the next page. However, if you want to learn how John Crittenden came to his conclusions and discoveries in *Blind Faith: Reverse Macular Degeneration Thru Diet & Nutrition*, I highly suggest you visit his website and read his book. He goes into great detail explaining the protocol and the methods he used to devise it. He also provides thorough descriptions of the vitamins, supplements, minerals, foods, and other interesting discoveries.

www.johncrittenden.com

Endnotes

[1] Crittenden, J. (2016). Blind faith: Reverse macular degeneration thru diet & nutrition. https://johncrittenden.com/

[2] What is the mechanism of Sodium Bicarbonate? https://synapse.patsnap.com/article/what-is-the-mechanism-of-sodium-bicarbonate

[3] Peskin, B. S. (2014). PEO Solution: Conquering Cancer, Diabetes and Heart Disease with Parent Essential Oil. Pinnacle Press. https://archive.org/details/peosolutionconqu0000bria

[4] Grounding: Exploring the Benefits of Earthing". WebMD, accessed December 30, 2024. https://www.webmd.com/balance/grounding-benefits

[5] The Critical Role of Growth Factors in Gastric Ulcer Healing: The Cellular and Molecular Mechanisms and Potential Clinical Implications. https://www.mdpi.com/2073-4409/10/8/1964

[6] What Is Vitamin Toxicity? https://www.verywellhealth.com/vitamin-toxicity-4776094

[7] Vitamin B12 levels in patients with retinal vein occlusion and their relation with clinical outcome: a retrospective study. https://link.springer.com/article/10.1007/s11739-021-02905-7

[8] How excess niacin may promote cardiovascular disease. https://www.nih.gov/news-events/nih-research-matters/how-excess-niacin-may-promote-cardiovascular-disease

[9] Is taking too much calcium unhealthy? https://www.health.harvard.edu/staying-healthy/is-taking-too-much-calcium-unhealthy

[10] Can You Overdose on Calcium? https://www.goodrx.com/well-being/supplements-herbs/too-much-calcium

[11] Pineal Gland. https://my.clevelandclinic.org/health/body/23334-pineal-gland

[12] 5 Functions of the Pineal Gland. https://www.healthline.com/health/pineal-gland-function

STEP 2: REPAIR THE EYE

[13] The Pineal Gland & Melatonin. https://www.drstevenlin.com/pineal-gland-melatonin/

[14] How Calcium Could Affect Your Brain. https://www.doctorshealthpress.com/how-calcium-could-affect-your-brain/

[15] The Calcium Connection: A Simple Nutrient Could Prevent Vision loss from Age-related Macular Degeneration. https://visionscienceacademy.org/the-calcium-connection-a-simple-nutrient-could-prevent-vision-loss-from-age-related-macular-degeneration/

[16] Inflammation in Retinal Vein Occlusion. https://onlinelibrary.wiley.com/doi/pdf/10.1155/2013/438412

[17] How Do Probiotics Survive Stomach Acid? https://guthealthimprovement.com/how-do-probiotics-survive-stomach-acid/

[18] National Research Council. (1989). Diet and health: Implications for reducing chronic disease risk. National Academies Press. https://nap.nationalacademies.org/catalog/19023/diet-and-health-implications-for-reducing-chronic-disease-risk-executive

My Daily Protocol

After four weeks of doing my version of the protocol, my eyesight improved to 20/100. Then, at eight weeks, it improved to 20/50, and finally, at twelve weeks, my vision was restored to 20/30.

Below is my exact daily regimen:

- Dissolve ½ teaspoon of baking soda in a small glass of water and drink it. Afterward, test your urine using pH balance strips, aiming for a pH level close to 8 (alkaline). Follow this cycle for eleven weeks, maintaining a routine of two weeks on and one week off.

- 2 tablets of Nature's Bounty Acidophilus Probiotic, taken in the morning and evening.

STEP 2: REPAIR THE EYE

- 3 tablets of Nature's Way Alive! Max3 Daily Adult Multivitamin.

- 3 tablets of Sports Research Evening Primrose Supplement from Cold Pressed Oil 1300mg.

- 2 tablets of Nature Made Extra Strength Flaxseed Oil 1400 mg.

- 1 tablet of Zhou Nutrition Garlic Supplement With Allicin, Extra Strength 5000 mcg.

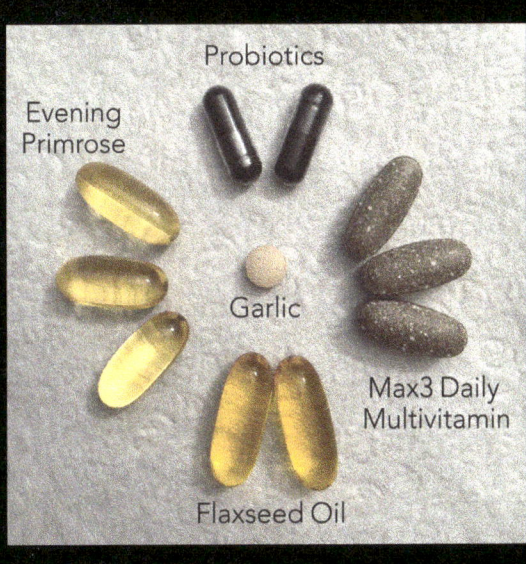

20

Step 3: Unblock the Blockage

Believe it or not, it took me almost a year before I realized that I wasn't doing anything to help my blocked vein. Ugh, in my naive innocence, I believed that the eye injections were tackling the problem. After all, wouldn't you expect my doctors to communicate and have a well-thought-out plan for my health issue? Sadly, they didn't. In America, except for smoking and drinking, most professional doctors and hospitals do not consider a patient's diet or lifestyle choices, which often account for many health issues.

Annoyed with myself for not figuring this out sooner, I took a moment to reflect

STEP 3: UNBLOCK THE BLOCKAGE

and remind myself that CRVO is called an eye stroke for a reason. Then, the memory of the ophthalmologist with the high-pitched laugh came rushing back. I remembered her saying, "There's a good chance that you have a blockage elsewhere in your body."

Thankfully, she was wrong about that, too. However, with no signs of heart disease, I didn't really know where to start to figure out the best way to unblock the blockage or if it was even possible to do so.

Is it possible to unblock a clogged artery?

The answer is yes. Heart disease patients routinely clear their blockages with the help of medications, surgeries, lifestyle changes, and other methods[4]. Even more exciting was the news that CRVO patients aren't left out in the cold. While the methods may differ from those used for heart disease, they too can manage and potentially unblock their occlusions[5].

Disappointingly, the options for unblocking CRVO were the usual suspects: anti-VEGF injections, laser surgery, steroids, and lifestyle changes. Yet, it was that last one that leaped off the page and grabbed my attention.

Lifestyle Changes

With everything in life, adopting healthier habits and behaviors can positively impact your overall well-being and reduce the risk of various health issues. Here are some key lifestyle changes that can positively impact your eye health and CRVO condition:

- Healthy Diet: Eating a diet rich in fruits, vegetables, and omega-3 fatty acids can help maintain good eye health. Foods like leafy greens, carrots, and fish are particularly beneficial[6].

STEP 3: UNBLOCK THE BLOCKAGE

- Regular Exercise: Physical activity improves blood circulation, which can help deliver essential nutrients to your eyes. It also reduces the risk of conditions like diabetes and high blood pressure, which can affect your vision[6].

- Quit Smoking: Smoking increases the risk of cataracts, age-related macular degeneration (AMD), and other eye diseases. Quitting smoking can significantly improve your eye health[6].

- Protect Your Eyes from UV Rays: Wearing sunglasses with UV protection can help prevent damage from the sun's harmful rays, reducing the risk of cataracts and other eye conditions[6].

- Manage Screen Time: Prolonged screen time can cause digital eye strain. Follow the 20-20-20 rule: every 20 minutes, take a 20-second break and look at something 20 feet away[6].

- Get Enough Sleep: Adequate sleep is crucial for overall health, including eye health. Lack of sleep can lead to eye fatigue and dry eyes[6].

- Stay Hydrated: Drinking enough water helps maintain the moisture levels in your eyes, preventing dryness and irritation[6].

- Regular Eye Check-Ups: Routine eye exams can help detect and treat eye conditions early on, preventing further damage[6].

By implementing these lifestyle changes, you can help heal, protect, and maintain your vision. However, while this information made sense, it felt too generic. I was looking for a specific guide that would tell me exactly what steps to take, something similar to John's protocol. So, I explored further, looking for diets and other ways to unblock the blockages.

STEP 3: UNBLOCK THE BLOCKAGE

Once again, I turned on my computer to research eye stroke, CRVO, heart disease, and whether there were any natural methods to heal clogged arteries and remove plaque. I was searching for any information that confirmed it was possible and offered practical solutions.

To be honest, I was very disappointed at first. Every web article offered the same information. It almost felt like they were copying the text and changing a few words here and there. Then, a friend suggested I watch the documentary called *Forks Over Knives*, which explores the bold assertion that the majority, if not all, of the so-called "diseases of affluence" plaguing us can be managed—or even reversed—by ditching our current diet of animal-based and processed foods. The documentary was very promising. I found the concepts easy to understand and plausible, so I shifted my focus to my diet.

Dietary Changes

While I was researching, I also found that there are plenty of foods that can naturally unclog your arteries and improve arterial health, potentially reducing plaque buildup in the process. But first, I needed to understand what was going on.

What is plaque?

Plaque is a sticky, waxy substance that builds up inside the arteries, leading to a condition called atherosclerosis. It is composed of various materials, including[7]:

- Cholesterol: A type of fat found in your blood[7].
- Calcium: A mineral that can deposit in the arteries[7].
- Fatty Substances: Different types of fats that accumulate over time[7].
- Cellular Waste Products: Byproducts of cell metabolism[7].

- Fibrin: A protein involved in blood clotting[7].
- Inflammatory Cells: White blood cells and other immune system components that can contribute to plaque formation[7].

Over time, plaque buildup can narrow the arteries, restrict blood flow, and increase the risk of heart attacks and strokes. Maintaining a healthy diet and lifestyle can help manage and reduce plaque buildup.

How does plaque form in the eye:

Plaque formation in the eye, particularly in the retina, can occur through a process similar to atherosclerosis but with some unique aspects:

- Damage to the Blood Vessels: The process often begins with damage to the blood vessels in the retina. This damage can be caused by factors such as high blood pressure, smoking, high cholesterol, and diabetes[9].

- Cholesterol and Lipid Accumulation: Low-density lipoprotein (LDL) cholesterol, often referred to as "bad" cholesterol, can infiltrate the damaged blood vessels in the retina. Over time, cholesterol and other lipids accumulate, forming plaques[10].

- Plaque Formation: These plaques are sticky, waxy substances made up of fat, cholesterol, calcium, and other materials. As they build up, they narrow the blood vessels, restricting blood flow to the retina[11].

- Hollenhorst Plaques: Sometimes, plaques from other parts of the body can break free and travel to the retina, causing blockages known as Hollenhorst plaques. These can lead to sudden vision loss in one eye[11].

- Ocular Ischemic Syndrome: Severe plaque buildup in the carotid arteries can reduce blood flow to the eyes, leading to a condition called ocular ischemic syndrome. This can cause vision issues and eye pain[9].

STEP 3: UNBLOCK THE BLOCKAGE

Research suggests that maintaining a healthy lifestyle, including a balanced diet and regular exercise, can help reduce the risk of plaque formation in the eyes[10].

After diving deep into various web articles, I surmised that my blockage was likely due to plaque buildup. Even though not all heart disease stems from plaque accumulation, plaque buildup significantly contributes to many heart conditions. The veins in the eye are incredibly tiny, so it doesn't take much to obstruct them. Realizing this, I knew that I needed to focus on the foods I was eating.

Ugh, now came the fun part: changing my diet. As promising as the documentary Forks Over Knives was for clearing veins of plaque, switching to a plant-based diet was not easy to maintain for long periods. So, I researched heart-healthy diets. These diets include:

- Fruits and Vegetables: Aim to eat a wide variety of fruits and vegetables in different colors.

- Whole Grains: Choose whole grains like oats, brown rice, whole wheat bread, and quinoa over refined grains like white bread and white rice.
- Fiber: Whole grains are high in fiber, which can help lower cholesterol levels and improve heart health.
- Healthy Proteins: Lean cuts of meat, plant-based proteins, fish, and poultry.
- Healthy Fats: Unsaturated fats while limiting saturated and trans fats.
- Low Sodium: Minimize salt intake.
- Limit Added Sugars: Reduce consumption of sugary foods and beverages.

Overview of Popular Heart-Healthy Diets

The Mediterranean Diet: This diet is rich in fruits, vegetables, whole grains, and healthy fats like olive oil. It has been shown to improve heart health and reduce

STEP 3: UNBLOCK THE BLOCKAGE

plaque buildup. The Mediterranean Diet is popular in Blue Zones, areas of the world where people are known to live longer and lead healthier lifestyles.

The DASH Diet: This diet focuses on reducing sodium intake and emphasizes fruits, vegetables, whole grains, and lean proteins. It helps lower blood pressure and improve overall heart health, which can reduce the risk of plaque buildup in the arteries and possibly in the eyes.

The Vegetarian Diet: This diet excludes most animal products and focuses on fruits, vegetables, and plant-based proteins like nuts, beans, and lentils. It lowers LDL and total cholesterol levels, reducing the risk of atherosclerosis in the body and possibly in the eyes.

In her web article "39 Foods That Unclog Arteries," Veronica Rouse, a registered dietitian (MAN, RD, CDE), uncovers the dangers of clogged arteries, which can lead to heart attacks and strokes [19]. She reveals that the common culprits are poor sleep, stress, lack of exercise, and an unhealthy diet. Rouse suggests that a wealth of evidence supports the benefits of a diet low in added sugars, refined grains, and trans fats while being rich in plant and whole foods for heart and overall health. Below, I have summarized her insights and listed the 39 foods that can help keep your arteries clear[19].

Nutrients to Choose More Often

- Soluble Fiber: Found in whole grains, vegetables, and fruits, it helps manage blood sugar and cholesterol[19].

- Unsaturated Fats (PUFAs, Omega 3s): Found in fatty fish, flaxseed, chia seeds, walnuts, and canola oil is essential for heart health[19].

- Antioxidants: Found in vegetables, fruits, nuts, and whole grains, they protect the body from free radicals and help keep the arteries clear[19].

STEP 3: UNBLOCK THE BLOCKAGE

Nutrients to Choose Less Often

- Saturated Fats: Found in animal fats, butter, and palm oil, they have been found to increase LDL cholesterol and heart disease risk[19].

- Processed Foods: High in sugar, salt, and trans fats, they provide empty calories with no nutritional benefits[19].

39 Foods That Unclog Arteries:

1) Garlic: Lowers blood pressure and cholesterol, improves CRP and CAC levels, reducing atherosclerosis risk[19].

2) Chia Seeds: Rich in omega-3s, lowers total cholesterol and raises HDL cholesterol[19].

3) Flaxseeds: Lowers blood pressure and cholesterol and are high in soluble fiber[19].

4) Olive Oil: Contains MUFAs (Monounsaturated Fatty Acids) and polyphenols, lowers LDL, and raises HDL cholesterol[19].

5) Green Tea: Rich in antioxidants, reduces inflammation, and improves cholesterol levels[19].

6) Tofu: Lowers LDL cholesterol and contains isoflavones (antioxidants), reducing atherosclerosis risk[19].

7) Salmon: High in omega-3s. Two servings per week are recommended for heart health[19].

8) Sardines: Rich in omega-3s and potassium, lowers blood pressure[19].

9) Anchovies: Contain a high amount of omega-3s and selenium, providing antioxidants that lower heart disease risk[19].

10) Mackerel: High in omega-3s, lowers LDL cholesterol, and raises HDL cholesterol[19].

STEP 3: UNBLOCK THE BLOCKAGE

11) Turmeric: High in curcumin, lowers inflammation, and prevents LDL oxidation[19].

12) Walnuts: Rich in PUFAs (Polyunsaturated Fatty Acids), fiber, minerals, and vitamins, they lower cholesterol and reduce the risk of heart disease[19].

13) Almonds: High in healthy fats, potassium, vitamins E and B, lowers LDL cholesterol, and improves HDL levels[19].

14) Avocado Oil: High in healthy fats, raises HDL levels, and promotes heart health[19].

15) Barley: Rich in beta-glucan (soluble fiber), lowers cholesterol levels[19].

16) Oats: Contain soluble and insoluble fiber and help manage blood sugar and cholesterol levels[19].

17) Strawberries: Rich in vitamin C and antioxidants, lowers LDL oxidation and inflammation[19].

18) Chickpeas: Contain a high amount of protein and soluble fiber, regulate cholesterol levels, and are heart-healthy[19].

19) Lentils: High in protein, fiber, potassium, and magnesium, lower blood pressure, and clean arteries.

20) Apples: Lower risk for clogged arteries, stroke, and LDL cholesterol due to flavonoids and fiber in the skin[19].

21) Pistachios: Manage blood sugar and lower cholesterol, inflammation, and oxidative stress due to fiber, antioxidants, and healthy fats[19].

22) Watermelon: Rich in fiber, vitamins, and lycopene, lowers LDL, increases HDL, and prevents plaque formation[19].

23) Beets: High in antioxidants, fiber, potassium, and magnesium, lower LDL oxidation and blood pressure, and improve arteries[19].

STEP 3: UNBLOCK THE BLOCKAGE

24) Asparagus: Lowers blood pressure and risk for hypertension and atherosclerosis, rich in potassium and vitamin C[19].

25) White Potatoes: Rich in vitamin C, fiber, and potassium. They lower inflammation and manage cholesterol and blood pressure[19].

26) Sweet Potatoes: Full of vitamins A, C, E, fiber, protein, and potassium, manage blood sugar and cholesterol levels[19].

27) Red Grapes: Rich in flavonoids like resveratrol, reduce platelet aggregation and LDL oxidation, lowering heart disease risk[19].

28) Ginger: Lowers inflammation and platelet aggregation, provides antioxidants, and is often used in traditional medicine[19].

29) Cinnamon: Manages sugar levels and blood pressure and lowers the risk for diabetes, hypertension, and atherosclerosis[19].

30) Tomatoes: Contain lycopene, lower blood pressure, and LDL cholesterol, and are versatile in cooking[19].

31) Broccoli: Contains quercetin, lowers inflammation and LDL oxidation, and is rich in calcium and folate[19].

32) Onions: Contain quercetin, lower LDL oxidation, blood pressure, and hypertension risk[19].

33) Sofrito: A sauce made of tomato, olive oil, onion, and garlic. This mixture contains lycopene and beta-carotene and reduces inflammation[19].

34) Spinach: Full of vitamins and minerals, produces nitric oxide, opens arteries, and lowers blood pressure[19].

35) Oranges: Rich in vitamins A and E, antioxidants, lower oxidative stress, LDL cholesterol, and hypertension risk[19].

36) Cranberries: Rich in anthocyanins, prevent LDL oxidation, fight free radicals, and are versatile in meals.

STEP 3: UNBLOCK THE BLOCKAGE

37) Pomegranate: Contains punicalagin, prevents oxidative stress and inflammation, and seeds can be added to various meals[19].

38) Avocado: Rich in potassium, magnesium, and soluble fiber. Increases HDL, reduces inflammation, and manages blood pressure[19].

39) Soy Milk: Contains soy protein and isoflavones, lowers LDL cholesterol, and reduces atherosclerosis risk[19].

By understanding these dietary recommendations and incorporating heart-healthy foods into your daily routine, you can proactively maintain arterial health, reduce the risk of further complications from CRVO, and help unblock the blockage.

Personally, I found it helpful to write down the foods I liked from these types of lists and then incorporate them into my meals. You might have noticed that multiple foods offer the same type of benefits, so if you don't like salmon, like me, you can find another type of fish or food that has the same nutrients. By doing so, these dietary changes become more enjoyable and easier to incorporate.

A Controversial Discovery

So, did changing my diet have any effect on my CRVO condition? Absolutely. Within a year, my eye condition improved, as did the numbers on my fundus photos. My doctor gradually extended the interval between my Eylea injections from every 4 to 6 weeks to every 7 to 10 weeks, spanning from the fall of 2018 to the fall of 2022. But let's be real—there was no instant gratification. It was a slow and unsteady journey, one where I occasionally stumbled and succumbed to greasy, unhealthy temptations. Yet, for the most part, I kept to a healthy diet.

STEP 3: UNBLOCK THE BLOCKAGE

However, in January 2023, everything shifted. One morning, after making eggs for breakfast, I had an epiphany. As I cleaned my plate, I struggled to remove the stubborn, sticky, dried yolk. It made me realize that if plaque were just as sticky, unblocking my eye could take a very long time. So, I searched my brain for things that remove sticky substances, and rubbing alcohol popped into my head. I've used it plenty of times to remove gooey residues from clothing, carpets, and other things.

Later that evening, I woke in the middle of the night wondering if folks in Italy who drank red wine with dinner every day suffered much from heart disease or plaque buildup. I grabbed my laptop and researched it. There were many positive articles on the benefits, so the following day, I contemplated whether or not I should give wine a shot.

Is wine good for the heart?

Yes, red wine, when consumed in limited amounts, has long been considered heart-healthy. Studies have shown that moderate red wine consumption is associated with a lower risk of cardiovascular disease and plaque buildup. This is due to the alcohol and antioxidants, particularly polyphenols like resveratrol, found in red wine. These substances may help prevent coronary artery disease by increasing levels of high-density lipoprotein (HDL) cholesterol and protecting against cholesterol buildup[17].

In a large research meta-analysis of 13 studies involving over 200,000 patients, red wine intake reduced the risk of plaque buildup in the arteries (atherosclerosis) by 37%[18]. This suggests that moderate consumption of red wine, a glass or two per day, may help prevent heart disease and reduce high blood pressure. However, these benefits are not 100% conclusive[18].

STEP 3: UNBLOCK THE BLOCKAGE

While the links between red wine and fewer heart attacks are not fully understood, antioxidants in red wine might help protect blood vessels, reduce low-density lipoprotein (LDL) cholesterol, and prevent blood clots[17]. However, research results on resveratrol are mixed, with some studies showing it may lower the risk of inflammation and blood clotting, while others do not[17].

Resveratrol is found in the skin of grapes used to make wine, as well as in peanuts, blueberries, and cranberries. Drinking grape juice or eating these foods might provide similar benefits without consuming alcohol[17]. Moderate consumption of any type of alcohol has been shown to help the heart by raising HDL cholesterol, preventing blood clots, and preventing artery damage from high LDL cholesterol levels[17]. However, excessive alcohol consumption can lead to numerous health problems, including high blood pressure, liver disease, certain cancers, and heart failure. This was a controversial subject for me because alcoholism runs in my family, and almost all of the articles mentioned that drinking wine every day could lead to it. Yet, I also had a lot of Italians in my family who drank wine every day with dinner and didn't suffer from the disease.

So, after all my reading and debating the dangers, I decided to give it a try. I had one rule that I promised myself I wouldn't break, and that was that I would only drink wine when I was eating dinner. That's because when you consume alcohol with food, it slows down the absorption of alcohol into your bloodstream[16]. Food in your stomach keeps the alcohol there longer, preventing it from quickly entering your bloodstream and making you feel intoxicated[16]. As a result, your blood-alcohol levels rise more slowly and don't get as high as they would on an empty stomach[16].

Additionally, having food in your stomach can help reduce the risk of a hangover and lighten the load on your liver, as the enzyme alcohol dehydrogenase (ADH) in your stomach can begin metabolizing the alcohol before it reaches your liver[16].

The Results

To my amazement, after just 8 weeks of enjoying 4 to 10 ounces of wine with dinner each night, my fundus photos showed remarkable improvement. At my next eye appointment, 8 weeks later, the results were even better. By the following visit, my numbers had surpassed all expectations. As my ophthalmologist peered into my eye through a slit lamp, he exclaimed, "Wow, it's like your body is trying to heal itself." I shared with him my nightly wine ritual. Intrigued, he encouraged me to continue.

Since then, my results have continued to improve to the point where I am now receiving injections every 12 to 15 weeks, depending on whether or not I had a blood leakage. I should note that I have had two minimal eye leaks in the past year, mainly because I've been pushing myself harder at the gym with a personal trainer, trying to get in shape and lose weight.

On the bright side, wine can make every meal taste better, and a pleasant buzz can be quite delightful. However, it comes with its own set of drawbacks. I've gained 10 pounds and struggle to lose weight. Wine can make you drowsy, and my sleep has been more restless than ever, leading me to occasionally take sleep aids—which aren't great either. Like other forms of alcohol, wine disrupts REM sleep, leading to fragmented and less restorative rest[20]. Experts recommend avoiding alcohol at least 3 hours before bed to minimize its impact on sleep quality[20]. Fortunately, I've managed to avoid slipping into alcoholism, which was my biggest worry. Even more promising is that incorporating wine has turned out to be a surprisingly effective ally in the recovery of my eyesight, which I plan to continue in a healthy way.

STEP 3: UNBLOCK THE BLOCKAGE

Unblock the Blockage Summary

After writing this chapter, it becomes evident to me that healing CRVO requires much more than just injections to treat the condition. Vision loss from retinal vein occlusions affects every aspect of life, including reading, writing, driving, performing daily chores, and even self-care. For reasons that stump me, many doctors in the United States and the health industry as a whole overlook the critical impact of diet, exercise, and lifestyle choices on eye health when crafting treatment plans[22]. Instead, they often zero in on treatment over prevention or cure—a bit like trying to extinguish fires without considering fire safety measures. It's hard to solve problems you don't yet have, right? Plus, tracking diet and lifestyle changes can be tricky, and patients often resist. Yet, these elements are vital. For example, a Mediterranean diet has been linked to a reduced risk of conditions like diabetic retinopathy[22]. For a fresh perspective, check out Outlive by Peter Attia, MD. He paints a compelling picture of Medicine 3.0, moving beyond the treatment-centric framework of Medicine 2.0 towards a more preventative approach[21].

Endnotes:

[1] Is It Possible to Unclog Your Arteries? https://www.healthline.com/health/heart-disease/how-to-unclog-arteries

[2] The #1 Way to Unclog Your Arteries Naturally, According to Cardiologists. https://parade.com/health/how-to-unclog-arteries-naturally-according-to-cardiologists

[3] How to Clean Your Arteries: Food and Lifestyle Changes to Unclog Arteries. https://www.doctorshealthpress.com/natural-foods-to-unclog-your-arteries/

[4] How to Treat Blocked Veins. https://www.wikihow.com/Treat-Blocked-Veins

[5] Central Retinal Vein Occlusion (CRVO). https://www.nei.nih.gov/learn-about-eye-health/eye-conditions-and-diseases/central-retinal-vein-occlusion-crvo

[6] How Your Lifestyle Affects Your Eye Health. https://billingseyedocs.com/eye-care/how-your-lifestyle-affects-your-eye-health/

[7] Can we reduce plaque buildup in arteries? https://www.health.harvard.edu/heart-health/can-we-reduce-vascular-plaque-buildup

[8] Verma, R. (2023). Plaque Formation: How it Develops and what you can do about it. Interventional Cardiology Journal, 2471-8157.

[9] Ocular Ischemic Syndrome. https://my.clevelandclinic.org/health/diseases/25205-ocular-ischemic-syndrome

STEP 3: UNBLOCK THE BLOCKAGE

[10] What Causes Plaque in the Eye? | Eye Health Unveiled. https://wellwisp.com/what-causes-plaque-in-the-eye/

[11] Hollenhorst Plaques. https://my.clevelandclinic.org/health/diseases/25136-hollenhorst-plaques

[12] 7 Bilberry Benefits (incl. Eye Health) + Side Effects & Dosage. https://supplements.selfdecode.com/blog/bilberry/

[13] What Is Garlic Extract? | Nature's Potent Remedy. https://wellwisp.com/what-is-garlic-extract/

[14] Red Wine and Your Heart. https://www.ahajournals.org/doi/10.1161/01.cir.0000151608.29217.62

[15] Light-to-Moderate Wine Consumption Tied to Lower Cardiovascular Disease Risk. https://www.msn.com/en-my/food-and-drink/beverages/light-to-moderate-wine-consumption-tied-to-lower-cardiovascular-disease-risk/ar-AA1wbHKt

[16] For Maximum Health Benefits, Have Your Wine with a Meal. https://www.winespectator.com/articles/for-maximum-health-benefits-have-your-wine-with-a-meal

[17] Red wine and resveratrol: Good for your heart? https://www.mayoclinic.org/diseases-conditions/heart-disease/in-depth/red-wine/art-20048281

[18] Red Wine: Is it Good for Your Heart? https://blog.nasm.org/nutrition/red-wine-good-heart?fbclid=IwZXh0bgNhZW0CMTEAAR2Sllsv3-vMu8euRrQTKj26zX7mUxfSAwC2NyVvpbqMFmgCh8cMlPHRXTg_aem_eA9q4CSsbdb4fKX6sL1w7A

[19] 39 Foods That Unclog Arteries. https://theheartdietitian.com/foods-that-unclog-arteries/

[20] Alcohol and Sleep. https://www.sleepfoundation.org/nutrition/alcohol-and-sleep

[21] Outlive: The Science & Art of Longevity. https://peterattiamd.com/outlive/

[22] Effects and Mechanism of Diet, Exercise and Lifestyle on Eye Health and Diseases. https://www.frontiersin.org/research-topics/63941/effects-and-mechanism-of-diet-exercise-and-lifestyle-on-eye-health-and-diseases

FINAL THOUGHTS

21

Conclusion

According to the website Europe PMC (europepmc.org), Retinal Vein Occlusions are on the rise globally. Now more than ever, there's a growing urgency for a cure or effective treatment to support CRVO survivors in maintaining, restoring, or regaining their vision. In this book, I delve into the nature of the condition, its causes, and the current medical treatments available. Additionally, I share my journey, detailing the steps I took to reclaim my vision and heal my eyesight.

CONCLUSION

In this final chapter, I will document the exact dates that reveal whether I experienced a blood leak, received an injection, or introduced new elements such as the protocol, dietary changes, and exercise. I'll also share my final thoughts on this journey.

Injection Timeline and Treatment Progress

2016

- 09/21/16: ***My first injection of Avastin.***
- 09/21/16 - 10/19/16: 4wks (leak, injection)
- 10/19/16 - 11/16/16: 4wks (leak, injection)
- 11/16/16 - 12/28/16: 6wks (BAD LEAK, injection)

2016 Summary: In 2016, I received Avastin injections every four weeks. However, from November to December, my doctor extended the interval to six weeks, and unfortunately, my eye's condition worsened, with leakage increasing significantly.

2017

- 12/28/16 - 01/26/17: 4wks (BAD LEAK, injection)
- 03/16/17 - 04/13/17: 4wks (BAD LEAK, injection)
- 04/13/17 - 05/15/17: 4wks (BAD LEAK, injection)
- 05/15/17 - 06/19/17: 4wks (leak, injection, **I began John's protocol**)
- 06/19/17 - 07/13/17: 4wks (**no leak**, injection)
- 07/13/17 - 08/24/17: 4wks (**no leak**, injection)
- 08/24/17 - 09/25/17: 4wks (**no leak, and I completed the protocol**, injection, **switched to Eylea**)
- 09/25/17 - 11/06/17: 6wks (BAD LEAK, injection, **restarted the protocol**)
- 11/06/17 - 12/18/17: 6wks (**no leak**, injection)

2017 Summary: In May 2017, I started John's protocol, switching to Eylea injections in August. Initially, the injections were administered every four weeks until September, after which the frequency was extended to every six weeks. This new protocol led to an improvement in my eye's condition, with fewer leaks occurring, even while I maintained a gym routine three times weekly.

CONCLUSION

2018

- 12/18/17 - 02/05/18: 7wks (BAD LEAK, injection)
- 02/05/18 - 03/19/18: 6wks (*no leak*, injection)
- 03/19/18 - 04/30/18: 6wks (BAD LEAK, injection)
- 04/30/18 - 07/11/18: 10wks (leak, injection, *I introduced dietary changes*)
- 07/11/18 - 08/27/18: 6wks (*no leak*, injection)
- 08/27/18 - 11/05/18: 10wks (leak, injection)
- 11/05/18 - 12/17/18: 6wks (*no leak*, injection)

2018 Summary: In April 2018, I adopted a heart-healthy diet by reducing my intake of sugar, salt, and fried foods. While I continued the protocol, I wasn't as strict with it, particularly with the use of baking soda. I would reintroduce it whenever I experienced bad leaks. The frequency of my injections ranged from every six to seven weeks. As a result of these changes, my eye's condition improved, and the leaks became milder.

2019

- 12/17/18 - 02/18/19: 9wks (**no leak**, injection)
- 02/18/19 - 04/18/19: 8wks (**no leak, NO injection**)
- 04/18/19 - 05/08/19: 3wks (leak, injection)
- 05/08/19 - 07/11/19: 9wks (**no leak**, injection)
- 07/11/19 - 09/16/19: 9wks (minor leak, injection)
- 09/16/19 - 11/18/19: 9wks (minor leak, injection)

2019 Summary: In 2019, I continued with the protocol and dietary changes, which resulted in fewer eye leaks. When leaks did occur, they were very minor. Consequently, my doctor extended the interval between injections to every eight to nine weeks.

2020

- 11/18/19 - 02/03/20: 11wks (minor leak, injection)
- 02/03/20 - 04/27/20: 12wks (leak, injection)
- 04/27/20 - 06/15/20: 7wks (**no leak**, Injection)
- 06/15/20 - 08/03/20: 7wks (minor leak, injection)
- 08/03/20 - 09/21/20: 7wks (**no leak**, injection)
- 09/21/20 - 11/30/20: 10wks (minor leak, injection)

CONCLUSION

2020 Summary: In 2020, as my eye's condition improved significantly, my doctor experimented with extending the interval between injections from seven to twelve weeks. Although this caused some minor leakage, the encouraging news was that my vision was gradually improving.

2021

- 11/30/20 - 02/15/21: 11wks (minor leak, injection)
- 02/15/21 - 04/19/21: 9wks (**no leak**, injection)
- 04/19/21 - 07/19/21: 13wks (BAD LEAK, injection)
- 07/19/21 - 09/20/21: 9wks (**no leak**, injection)
- 09/20/21 - 11/18/21: 8wks (**no leak**, injection)

2021 Summary: In 2021, my CRVO condition showed significant improvement, and the leakage in my eye was largely subsiding. Consequently, my doctor continued to experiment with extending the interval between injections from eight to thirteen weeks.

2022

- 11/18/21 - 01/31/22: 10wks (minor leak, injection)
- 01/31/22 - 04/13/22: 10wks (minor leak, injection)
- 04/13/22 - 06/23/22: 10wks (**no leak**, injection)
- 06/23/22 - 09/08/22: 11wks (**no leak**, injection)
- 09/08/22 - 12/08/22: 13wks (BAD LEAK, injection)

2022 Summary: In 2022, my condition began to stabilize, and the leakage was minimal. The interval between injections remained steady at ten to eleven weeks.

2023

- 12/08/22 - 02/20/23: 10wks (**no leak**, injection, *I introduced wine with dinner*)
- 02/20/23 - 05/15/23: 12wks (minor leak, injection)
- 05/15/23 - 07/24/23: 10wks (**no leak**, injection)
- 07/24/23 - 10/16/23: 12wks (minor leak, injection)
- 10/16/23 - 01/04/24: 11wks (**no leak**, injection)

2023 Summary: In January 2023, I incorporated wine at dinner into my CRVO regimen. Within a few doctor's visits, my ophthalmologist extended the interval between injections to ten to twelve weeks.

CONCLUSION

2024

- 01/04/24 - 04/04/24: 13wks (minor leak, injection, *I started exercising with a trainer*)
- 04/04/24 - 07/17/24: 15wks (BAD LEAK, injection).
- 07/17/24 - 10/17/24: 13wks (minor leak, injection)
- 10/17/24 - 12/16/24: 8wks (*no leak*, injection)

2024 Summary: In 2024, my CRVO eye was doing exceptionally well until I overexerted myself at the gym in April, which set my healing process back a bit. However, overall, I only needed four injections that year, with intervals mostly ranging from thirteen to fifteen weeks. The last injection was administered earlier than usual because my doctor was going away for the holidays.

MY PROGRESS

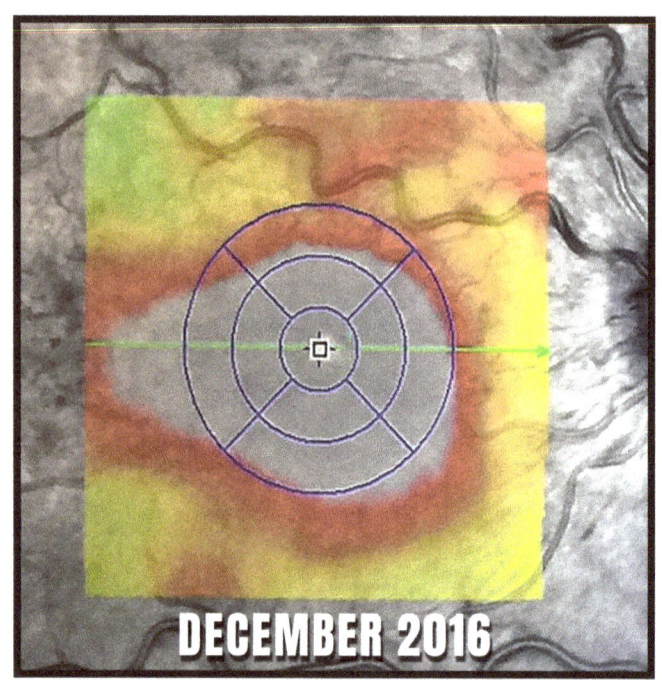

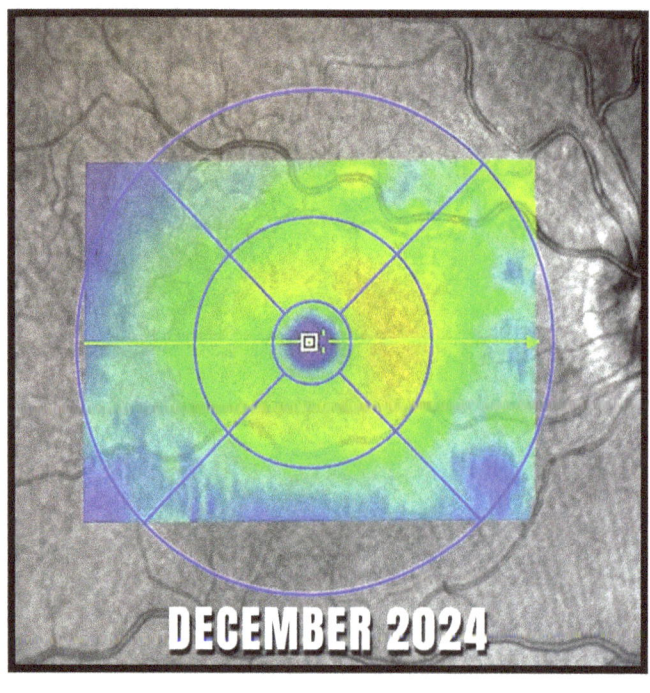

CONCLUSION

Reflections on
My CRVO Journey

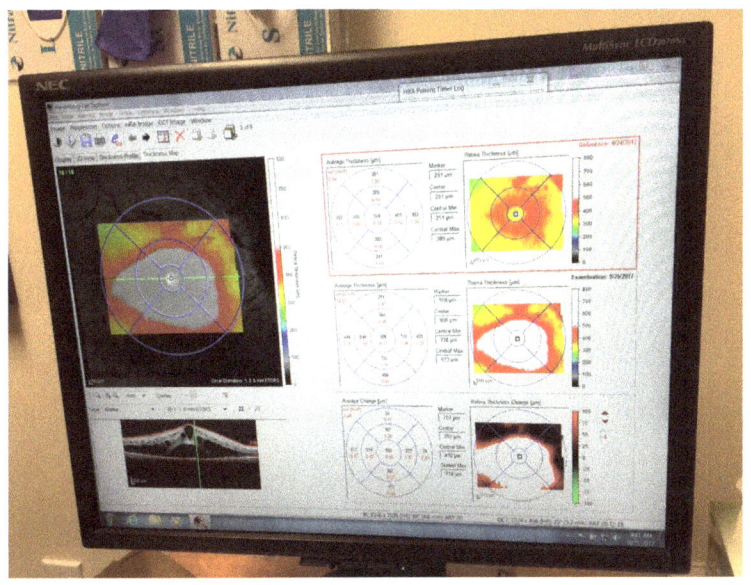

Upon examining my CRVO fundus photos from September 2016 to December 2024, it is evident that the injections significantly improved my condition. When present in the eye, the medication effectively prevented the abnormal blood vessels from leaking. However, it is also clear that it did not heal the eye itself.

Yet, with the help of John's protocol, my dietary changes, and the addition of 4 to 10 ounces of wine daily with dinner, the combination had an amazing impact on healing my condition and eye health.

Additionally, while reviewing the timeline between injections, I realized how inconsistent my doctor was with my follow-up appointments. The delay often caused bad eye leaks because the medicine had left my eye.

Another issue I wanted to highlight is how blood leakage from exercising can significantly set back your healing process. For example, when I hired a personal trainer in December 2023 to help me get in shape and lose weight, my eye leaked in April 2024. That leakage persisted throughout the year and finally settled down in December 2024. So, once again, be mindful of your blood pressure.

Parting Thoughts

It's interesting... I received my first injection in September 2016, then started following John's protocol in 2017, introduced dietary changes in 2018, and began the wine-with-dinner ritual in 2023. After eight long years, as I reflect on those key steps and the profound impact they had on healing my eye, I can't help but wonder: What if my doctors or the medical community had recommended something akin to John's protocol along with dietary changes from the very beginning? Could I have healed my CRVO within a year of my prognosis? My gut tells me yes, and that's why I wrote this.

My hope is that this book calms your fears and becomes a source of valuable insights, guiding you toward improving your condition and reclaiming your vision.

Best Wishes & Happy Healing
CRVO Survivor

22

Supplement Facts

Here are the supplement facts taken from the products themselves. This regimen is designed for eleven weeks, but I've continued taking the supplements and vitamins as I saw fit. The only exception to my daily routine is the baking soda, which I use less consistently since it's a temporary measure to make the body less acidic.

Below is my exact daily regimen:

- Dissolve ½ teaspoon of baking soda in a small glass of water and drink it. Afterward, test your urine using pH balance strips, aiming for a pH level close to 8 (alkaline). Follow this cycle for eleven weeks, maintaining a routine of two weeks on and one week off.

- 2 tablets of Nature's Bounty Acidophilus Probiotic, taken in the morning and evening.

- 3 tablets of Nature's Way Alive! Max3 Daily Adult Multivitamin.

- 3 tablets of Sports Research Evening Primrose Supplement from Cold Pressed Oil 1300mg.

- 2 tablets of Nature Made Extra Strength Flaxseed Oil 1400 mg.

- 1 tablet of Zhou Nutrition Garlic Supplement With Allicin, Extra Strength 5000 mcg.

Breakdown of the Components

SUPPLEMENT FACTS

1) Arm & Hammer Pure Baking Soda:

- Sodium Bicarbonate: 1 g, (no DV established)

2) Nature's Bounty Acidophilus Probiotic:

- Lactobacillus Acidophilus: 100 million CFU, (no DV established)
- Vegetable Cellulose: (no DV established)
- Vegetable Stearic Acid: (no DV established)
- Silica: - (no DV established)
- Vegetable Magnesium Stearate: (no DV established)

3) Nature's Way Alive! Max3 Potency Adult Complete Multivitamin:

- Vitamin A: 810 mcg, 300% DV
- Vitamin C: 900 mg, 333% DV
- Vitamin D3: 50 mcg, 83% DV

- Vitamin E: 100 mg, 222% DV
- Vitamin K: 120 mcg, 33% DV
- Thiamin: 20 mg, 556% DV
- Riboflavin: 20 mg, 512% DV
- Niacin: 100 mg, 208% DV
- Vitamin B6: 20 mg, 392% DV
- Folate: 400 mcg, 139% DV
- Vitamin B12: 80 mcg, 1,111% DV
- Biotin: 33 mcg, 37% DV
- Pantothenic Acid: 63 mg, 420% DV
- Choline: 30 mg, 2% DV
- Calcium: 325 mg, 8% DV
- Magnesium: 130 mg, 14% DV
- Zinc: 11 mg, 12% DV
- Selenium: 158 mcg, 158% DV
- Copper: 0.9 mg, 10% DV
- Manganese: 5.8 mg, 17% DV
- Molybdenum: 45 mcg, 5% DV

SUPPLEMENT FACTS

- Daily Greens™ Blend: Spirulina, Kelp, Barley grass, Blessed Thistle, Blue-Green Algae, Chlorella, Cilantro, Dandelion, Lemon Balm, Lemongrass, Nettle, Plantain, Wheat grass

- Orchard Fruits & Garden Veggies Blend: Apple, Pear, Cranberry, Raspberry, Strawberry, Carrot, Tomato, Spinach, Broccoli, Cabbage, Kale, Parsley, Peas, Onion, Garlic

- Mushroom Defense Blend: Shiitake, Maitake, Reishi, Turkey Tail

- Cardio Blend: Hawthorn Berry, Garlic, Ginkgo Biloba, Coenzyme Q10

- Digestive Enzyme Blend: Bromelain, Papain, Amylase, Lipase, Protease

- Omega Blend: Fish Oil, Flaxseed Oil, Borage Oil

- Lutein: 250 mcg

4) Sports Research Evening Primrose Oil:

- 1300 mg (no DV established)

5) Nature Made Flaxseed Oil:

- Alpha Linolenic Acid (Omega-3): 500 mg, 31% DV
- Linoleic Acid (Omega-6): (no DV established)
- Oleic Acid (Omega-9): (no DV established)
- Vitamin E: (no DV established)
- Gelatin: (no DV established)
- Glycerin: (no DV established)
- Water

6) Garlic Pills with Allicin:

- Allicin: 5000 mcg, (no DV established)
- Garlic (Allium sativum) Bulb Extract: 415 mg (Supplying 5,000 mcg [12,000 mcg/g] Allicin)

SUPPLEMENT FACTS

*Remember to monitor your acidity or alkalinity levels daily by testing your urine with pH balance strips.

JUST A NOTE: After four weeks of following my version of the protocol, my eyesight improved to 20/100. At eight weeks, it improved further to 20/50, and finally, at twelve weeks, my vision was restored to 20/30. I hope you experience the same success as I did.

Good Luck!

23

Helpful Links

- John Crittenden: https://johncrittenden.com/

- Book: BLIND FAITH: The Incredible Story of a Professional Artist Who Overcame Blindness Through Diet & Nutrition.

CRVO Support Groups

- Central Retinal Vein Occlusion Support (Google group): https://groups.google.com/g/crvo-support

- CRVO Support Group (Facebook group): https://www.facebook.com/groups/2301897780069475/

- Macular Society - Beating Macular Disease. Retinal vein occlusion (RVO): https://www.macularsociety.org/macular-disease/macular-conditions/retinal-vein-occlusion/

- Non-Ischemic CRVO Recovery (Google group): https://groups.google.com/g/crvo-support/c/iugUt8IDYIA

- Retinal Vein Occlusion - BRVO and CRVO companions (Facebook Group): https://www.facebook.com/groups/308659717252800/

www.ingramcontent.com/pod-product-compliance
Lightning Source LLC
Chambersburg PA
CBHW052028030426
42337CB00027B/4914